W9-CCC-044

Dr Ante Bilić
liječnik - stomatolog

EXERCISES IN DENTAL RADIOLOGY

VOLUME 1

INTRA-ORAL RADIOGRAPHIC INTERPRETATION

ROBERT P. LANGLAIS, B.A., D.D.S., M.S.

Assistant Professor, Department of Oral Diagnosis and
Radiology, Faculty of Dentistry, McGill University,
Montreal

MYRON J. KASLE, D.D.S., M.S.D.

Professor and Chairman, Department of Dental
Radiology, Indiana University School of Dentistry,
Indianapolis

W. B. SAUNDERS COMPANY   Philadelphia / London / Toronto

W. B. Saunders Company: West Washington Square
Philadelphia, PA 19105

1 St. Anne's Road
Eastbourne, East Sussex BN21 3UN, England

1 Goldthorne Avenue
Toronto, Ontario M8Z 5T9, Canada

Library of Congress Cataloging in Publication Data

Langlais, Robert P.

Intra-oral radiographic radiology.

(Exercises in dental radiology; v. 1)

1. Teeth — Radiography — Problems, exercises, etc.
   I. Kasle, Myron J., joint author.   II. Title
   III. Series. [DNLM: 1. Radiography, Dental — Examination
   questions WN18 L282e]

RK309.L34   617.6'07'572   77-79397

ISBN 0-7216-5624-2

Exercises in Dental Radiology — Volume 1

Intra-Oral Radiographic Interpretation   ISBN   0-7216-5624-2

© 1978 by W. B. Saunders Company.   Copyright under the International Copyright Union.
All rights reserved.   This book is protected by copyright.   No part of it may be reproduced,
stored in a retrieval system, or transmitted in any form or by any means, electronic, mechan-
ical, photocopying, recording, or otherwise, without written permission from the publisher.
Made in the United States of America.   Press of W. B. Saunders Company.   Library of
Congress catalog card number 77-79397

Last digit is the print number: 9   8   7   6

To our teachers—our students

FOREWORD

Dental radiology is the "Cinderella" of dentistry, and despite the fact that it is well taught in most dental schools, it is on the whole poorly learned by the average practicing dentist, although there are many who have substantial or even great interest in its pursuit. The quality of dental radiographic technique is, in general, equally poor, so that as a consequence, most dentists are unacquainted with the radiographic appearances of all but a few of the most common pathological processes that may occur in and about the teeth and jaws. As a rare consequence of this, serious or even grave outcomes occur for the patients.

Dental schools differ in their attitudes toward the value of radiology in dental education and practice, and some schools have no oral radiologist. This is detrimental not only to the education of the student but also to the standard of radiologic service within the institution, perhaps most noticeably in the department of surgery where maximal help is needed but is often not forthcoming.

Good textbooks exist, but readers have to be motivated to read them, and adequate motivation is often lacking once the student has graduated and entered practice. Most of these textbooks use a didactic approach, but this one of Drs. Langlais and Kasle is somewhat Socratic and is also highly imaginative, for alongside the many illustrations that have been selected for their pertinent contents, searching questions are asked that are designed to engender interest, to instruct, and to exercise the mind. As a similar format is used in examinations, students are indoctrinated to become familiar with this method. Answers are supplied that illuminate the information inherent in the selected radiographic illustrations. Imagination has been used in selecting appropriate illustrations and sensitive prescience in posing searching questions directed to educating the observer and student. Thus, student and practitioner can, if they wish, increase their knowledge of interpretative radiology.

Those who are interested in the propagation of knowledge owe a debt of gratitude to Drs. Langlais and Kasle for their industry and efforts in compiling this book. It is greatly to be hoped that they will reap where they have tilled and sowed.

H. M. WORTH, LL.D. Hon. Causa Toronto, F.R.C.P.(C.),
F.R.C.R., F.D.S., R.C.S. Eng.

PREFACE

The areas of oral diagnosis and radiology are basic to proper dental patient diagnosis and treatment planning. Visual clinical examination and correct radiographic interpretation correlated with the patient's history and appropriate laboratory values are all necessary to achieve excellence in patient diagnosis and treatment.

We have attempted herein to meet the needs of both students and practitioners with this question-and-answer format. Note that in many cases, certain laboratory values, significant data from the medical, dental, or social history, or the patient's symptoms are given. Use these clues to achieve first the differential diagnosis, and then, with the information given, try to arrive at a substantive working or final diagnosis. When the information contained in the radiographic picture is considered pathognomonic for a certain condition, then no further information other than the radiograph should be required to make the diagnosis. We have included exercises on the identification of normal landmarks as well as possible film artifacts. A knowledge of these areas is essential if accurate diagnosis of disease is to be made and must be acquired if one is to achieve continuing excellence in clinical technique. We have included exercises in the use of the "buccal object rule" because although the principle is simple, its application, if not understood, often generates confusion for the "student" of radiology. We hope that these exercises are the "practice that makes perfect" and will serve as a handy reference on occasions when the buccal object rule is to be used.

In making the differential diagnosis, be certain that the conditions that you select are defendable. In other words, if the lesion is five centimeters in diameter, do not select a lesion that rarely exceeds one centimeter. If the location is in the maxillary cuspid area, do not select a condition that usually occurs in the mandibular molar-ramus area. If the radiograph shows a multilocular radiolucency, do not include entities that are usually unilocular. Select the most commonly occurring lesions with their usual appearance, location, symptoms, and treatment.

The reader should keep in mind that the radiographs are mounted as if viewed from the outside, looking into the oral cavity. The convexity of the film identification dot is facing you.

Well, we hope that you enjoy testing yourself with these selected exercises. You may be pleasantly surprised to find that your knowledge is high; conversely, you may also learn how much you've forgotten! We think that learning should be fun, and we hope you enjoy this learning experience.

R. L.
M. K.

ACKNOWLEDGMENTS

The authors wish to express their appreciation to the following individuals for their assistance with this manuscript: Denyse Langlais for her constant support and encouragement and for typing the preliminary manuscript; Mr. Richard Scott, Director of Dental Illustrations, Indiana University School of Dentistry, and his staff, Mike Halloran and Alana Fears, for the illustrations; Dr. Rolando De Castro for the masterful artwork in Section 5; the following staff members of the Radiology Department of Indiana University School of Dentistry: Gail Williamson, R.D.H., Carol Ann Steinmetz, and Rosalie Pollack; and the following for allowing us to use certain radiographs:

Dr. Carson Mader	Figures 4–1, 4–15, 4–93
Dr. Sam Eitner	Figure 4–5
Dr. Tom McDavid	Figures 4–14, 4–16, 4–88
Dr. Monique Michaud	Figures 4–132, 4–150
Dr. William Goebel	Figure 4–141
Dr. Malcolm Boone II	Figures 4–119, 4–136
Dr. Stephen Bricker	Figures 4–79, 4–97
Dr. Robert Hampshire	Figure 4–16 (A, B, C)
Dr. Jim Cottone	Figure 4–165 (B, C)
Dr. David Blair	Figure 4–116

CONTENTS

SECTION 1

NORMAL ANATOMIC STRUCTURES

FIGURE 1–1

What entities are the arrows pointing at?

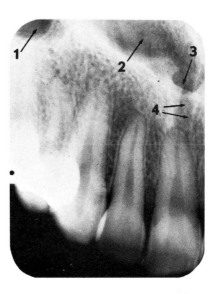

FIGURE 1–2

The arrows are pointing at what entities?

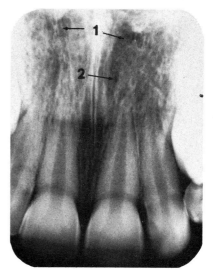

FIGURE 1–3

What is the common name used for this anatomic landmark, and what are the structures that make it up?

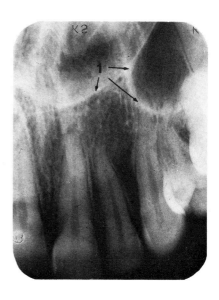

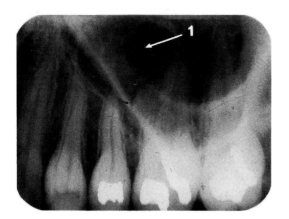

FIGURE 1-4

1. What does the round radiolucent area in this radiograph represent?

2. What could it be misdiagnosed as?

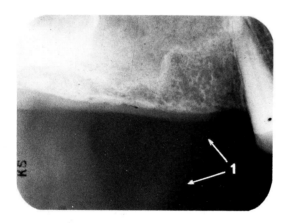

FIGURE 1-5

The border of what entity is indicated by the arrows?

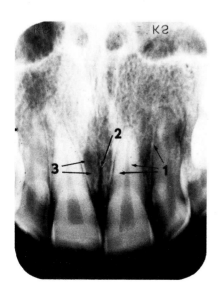

FIGURE 1-6

The arrows are pointing at what commonly recognized structures?

FIGURE 1-7

When the dentist wishes to see this structure the x-ray exposure should be decreased. What is this structure?

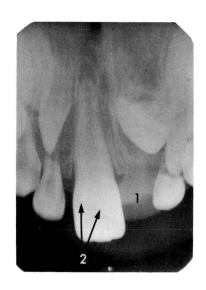

FIGURE 1-8

Entity 1 is commonly found in the wall of entity 2. Entity 3 is often seen outlining entity 2.

Name the entities indicated in this radiograph.

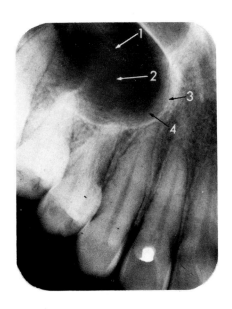

FIGURE 1-9

This view of the maxillary tuberosity area normally contains what entities?

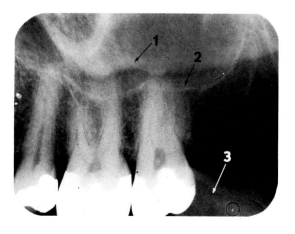

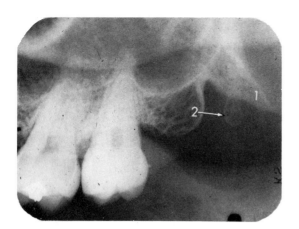

FIGURE 1–10

What do we see in this view?

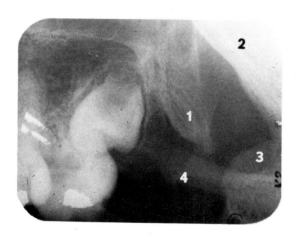

FIGURE 1–11

Viewing the maxillary tuberosity from an extremely posterior position gives one an opportunity to see structures not commonly visible on this intra-oral film. See if you can name them without looking at the answer page.

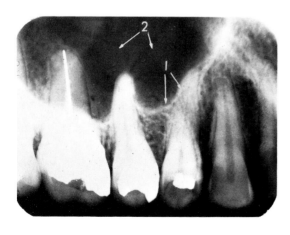

FIGURE 1–12

What entities does this periapical view show?

6

FIGURE 1-13

1. What is the radiolucent area seen between the maxillary lateral incisor and cuspid called?

2. What is it sometimes misdiagnosed as?

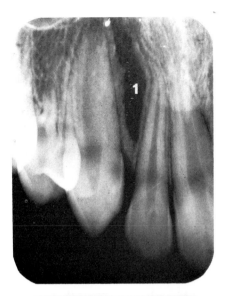

FIGURE 1-14

What radiographic images does this maxillary periapical view demonstrate?

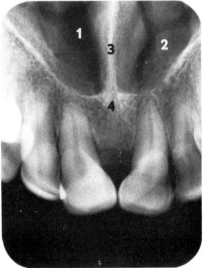

FIGURE 1-15

What does this radiograph demonstrate?

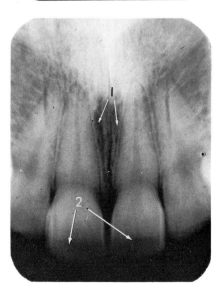

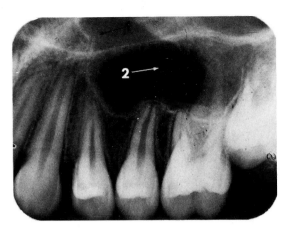

FIGURE 1–16

What do the arrows point at?

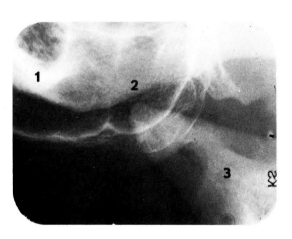

FIGURE 1–17

What do the images viewed in this radiograph of an edentulous maxilla represent?

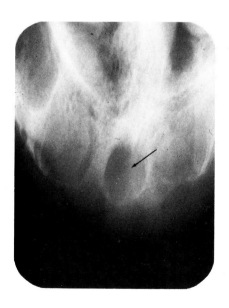

FIGURE 1–18

The arrow is pointing to a maxillary landmark that is sometimes incorrectly identified. What is the name of the landmark, and what is it sometimes incorrectly called?

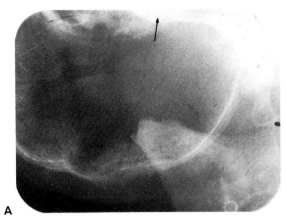

A

FIGURE 1–19

In radiograph *A*, the zygomatic process is seen at the top of the picture. In radiograph *B*, the zygomatic process is seen in the middle and to the right of the picture. Explain the differences in these two films.

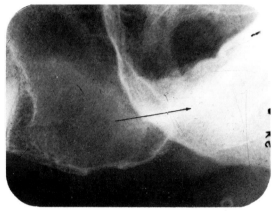

B

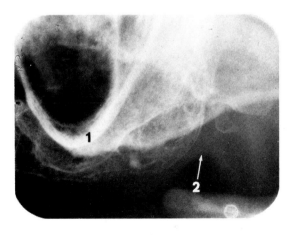

FIGURE 1–20

What anatomic landmarks does this view of an edentulous patient demonstrate?

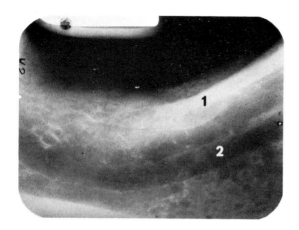

FIGURE 1-21

What are two commonly seen anatomic landmarks?

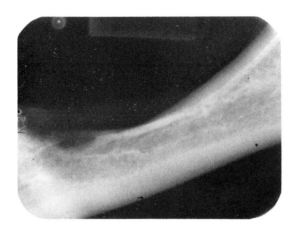

FIGURE 1-22

What is the radiolucency seen on the crest of the ridge?

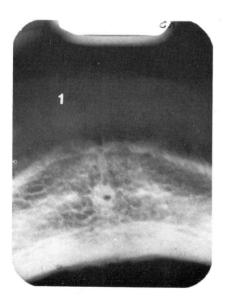

FIGURE 1-23

The first thing to do is to identify the area you're looking at. When you've done that identify (1) and the round radiopaque area in the center of the bone. What is the small radiolucency in the center of this round radiopaque area?

10

FIGURE 1-24

1. What does the radiolucency at the apex of the first bicuspid represent?

2. What does the radiolucent area apical to the first molar represent?

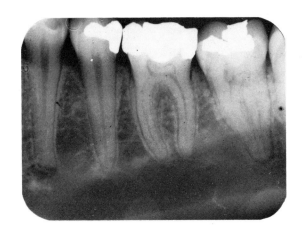

FIGURE 1-25

What are the vertical radiolucent lines viewed on this radiograph?

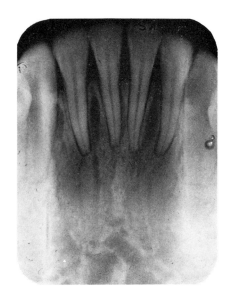

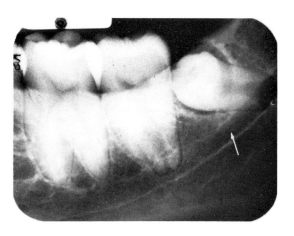

FIGURE 1-26

What is the arrow pointing at?

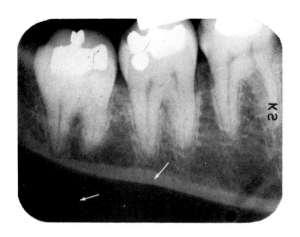

FIGURE 1-27

1. What does the upper arrow indicate the location of?
2. What does the lower arrow indicate the location of?

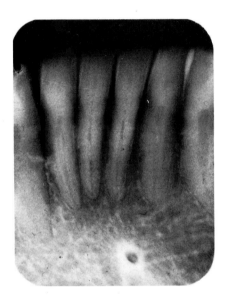

FIGURE 1-28

What is the round radiolucent area in the bone surrounded by a halo of radiopacity identified as?

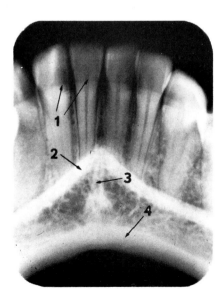

FIGURE 1-29

Beginning at the top, list the areas indicated by the arrows.

12

FIGURE 1–30

The arrows are pointing at an anatomic structure that is not usually seen on a periapical radiograph. What is this structure?

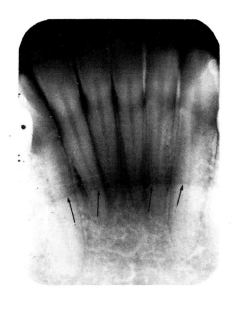

SECTION 2

FILM-HANDLING
AND
PROCESSING ERRORS

FIGURE 2–1

What is your explanation of the radio-lucency seen mainly in the cervical area of the maxillary cuspid and first bicuspid teeth? What causes this?

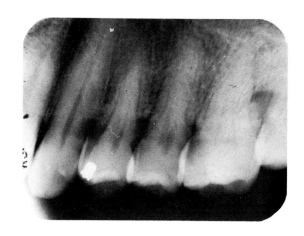

FIGURE 2–2

What term, coined by Dr. David F. Mitchell of Indiana University School of Dentistry, describes the film-handling error seen in this radiograph?

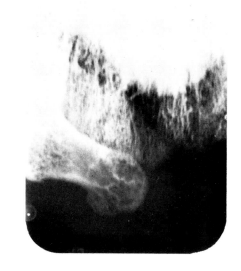

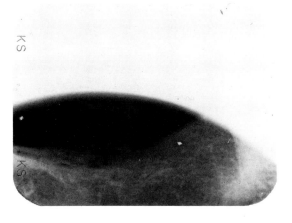

FIGURE 2–3

1. What exposure error was made here?
2. Identify the two small radiopaque spots seen on this film.

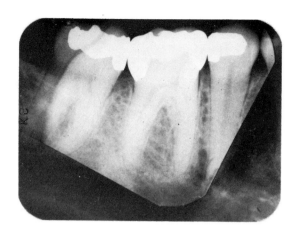

FIGURE 2-4

What film-handling error was made here?

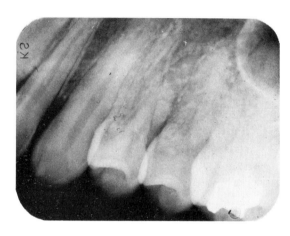

FIGURE 2-5

Why do the roots of the bicuspid teeth appear "fuzzed out"?

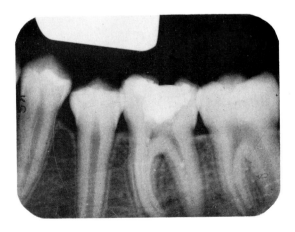

FIGURE 2-6

Name two possible causes for the inadequate periapical coverage.

FIGURE 2–7

How can a "blank" image such as this be produced?

FIGURE 2–8

What exposure error or errors may have been made here?

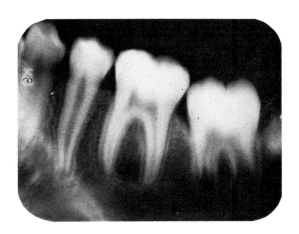

FIGURE 2–9

1. How would you describe the overall appearance of this radiograph?
2. How does this occur?

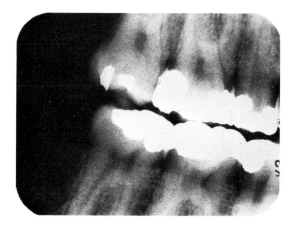

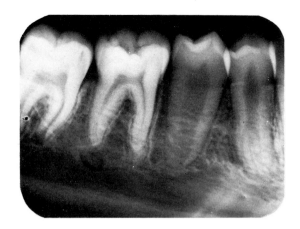

FIGURE 2-10

What processing solution can produce the artifact seen at the apex of the mandibular first molar?

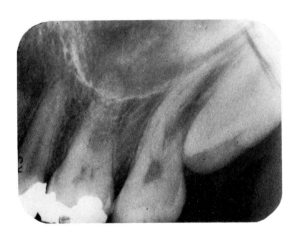

FIGURE 2-11

What film-handling error was made here?

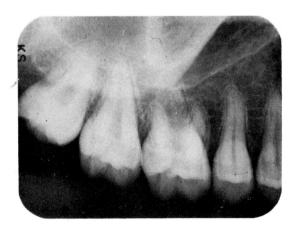

FIGURE 2-12

1. What exposure error was made?
2. What was the cause?

FIGURE 2–13

What film-handling error was made here?

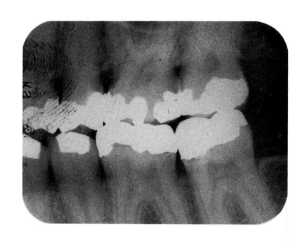

FIGURE 2–14

What processing solution may produce this artifact?

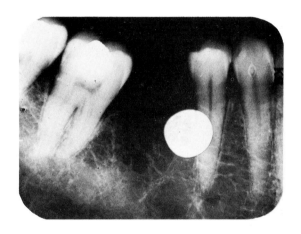

FIGURE 2–15

Now, tell us what exposure error was made here.

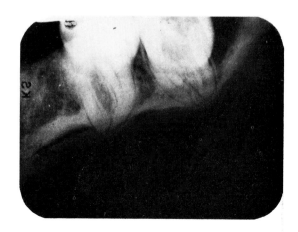

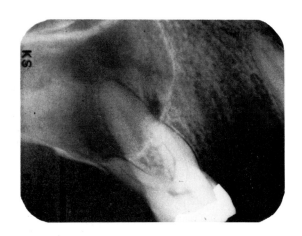

FIGURE 2-16

Why does the palatal root appear to be so much longer than the mesial buccal and distal buccal roots of this maxillary molar?

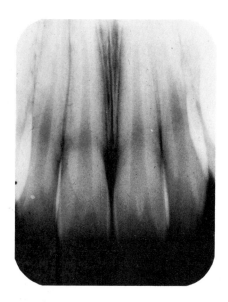

FIGURE 2-17

What error was made? Explain your answer.

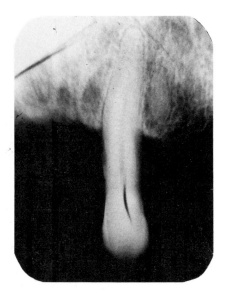

FIGURE 2-18

Can you name two film errors evident in this radiograph? Yes, you can. Try.

FIGURE 2–19

What exposure error has been made here? How?

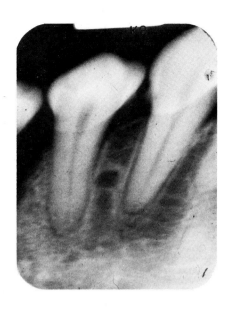

FIGURE 2–20

List some reasons why this film is too light.

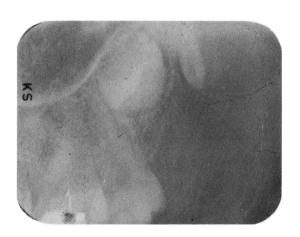

FIGURE 2–21

1. What anatomic structure is superimposed over the entire crown and root of the maxillary molar?
2. How did this superimposition occur?

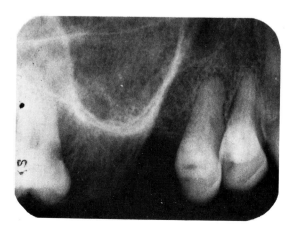

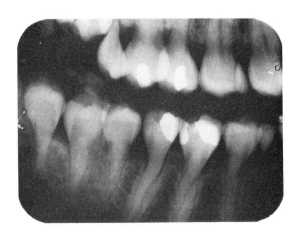

FIGURE 2-22

What exposure error was made?

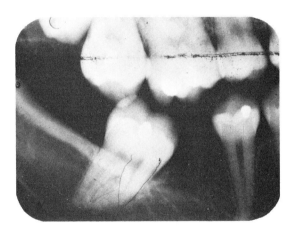

FIGURE 2-23

What do you suppose produced the horizontal black line across the crowns of the maxillary teeth in this radiograph developed by automatic film-processing methods?

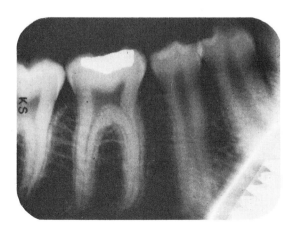

FIGURE 2-24

Give a commentary on the white line seen in the lower right-hand corner of this film.

FIGURE 2–25

List possible reasons why this film is too dark.

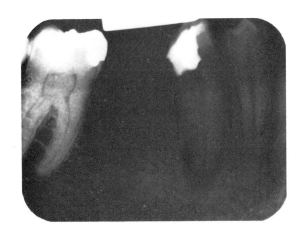

FIGURE 2–26

What technical error was made? How?

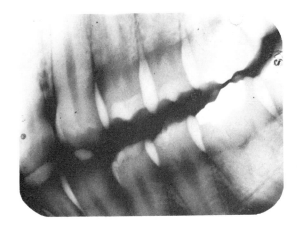

FIGURE 2–27

What film-handling error produced this radiopaque artifact over the second molar?

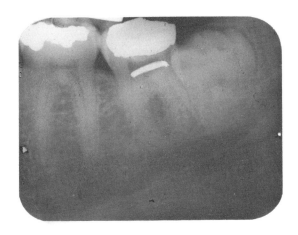

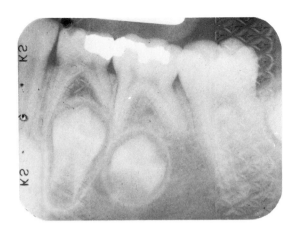

FIGURE 2–28

What film-handling error was made?

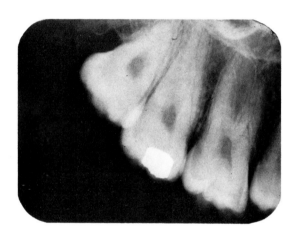

FIGURE 2–29

Why were the apices of the second and third maxillary molars missed?

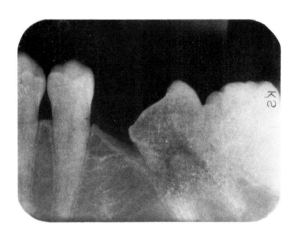

FIGURE 2–30

What processing error was made?

FIGURE 2-31

List possible reasons why this film was fogged.

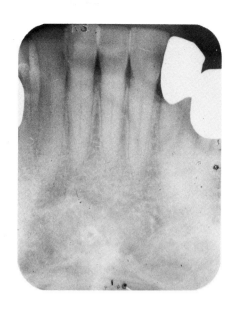

FIGURE 2-32

Give your differential diagnosis of the condition represented by the radiopaque portion of the periapical radiolucency seen in this radiograph. Include possible artifacts.

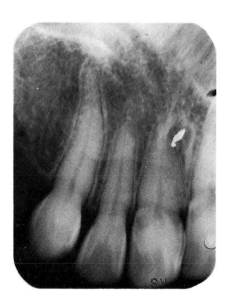

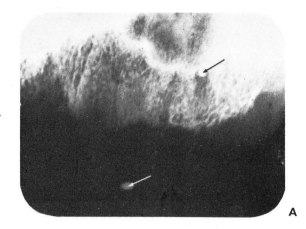

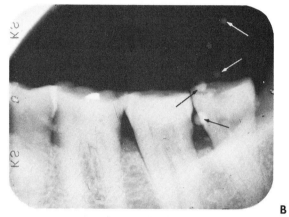

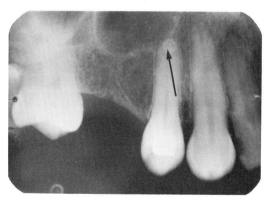

A

B

C

FIGURE 2–33

The radiopaque circular areas in these three radiographs are all of different origins. What is your list of possible causes of these opacities (arrows)?

FIGURE 2-34

What film-processing artifact is present here?

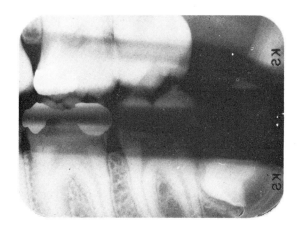

FIGURE 2-35

1. What does the radiolucent line with radiopaque borders in the upper right corner of the film represent?

2. What does the radiopaque line in the lower right corner of the film represent?

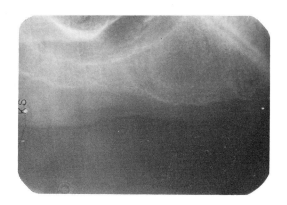

FIGURE 2-36

1. What anatomic structure superimposed on the maxillary antrum is causing the sinus to appear cloudy, as if fluid filled?

2. What exposure error produced this effect?

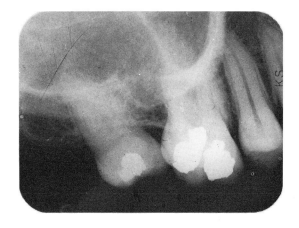

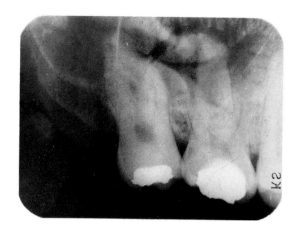

FIGURE 2-37

After processing of this radiograph in solutions at 90°F, the film was rinsed under the cold-water tap. What term is used to describe the damaged emulsion produced by this film-processing error?

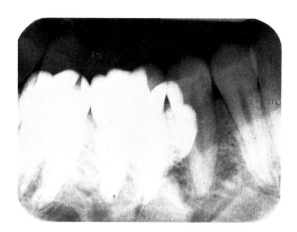

FIGURE 2-38

What film-handling error was made?

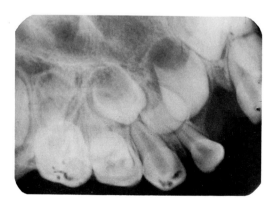

FIGURE 2-39

What artifact, which mimics enamel hypoplasia, is present in this radiograph of deciduous teeth?

FIGURE 2–40

The artifact seen on this radiograph resembles a fistulous tract. What is this artifact?

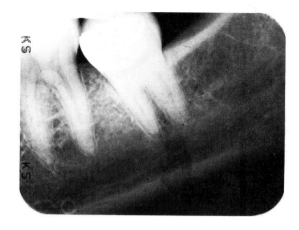

FIGURE 2–41

What film-handling or processing errors are evident here?

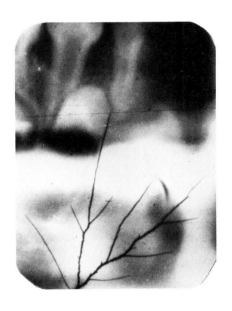

FIGURE 2–42

What artifact is present here?

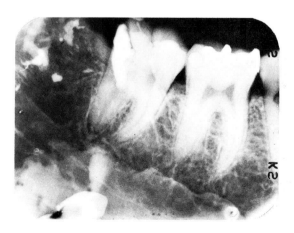

SECTION 3

IDENTIFICATION OF MATERIALS

AND

FOREIGN OBJECTS

FIGURE 3–1

1. What materials could have been used to restore the mesial of the central incisors?

2. What materials could have been used to restore the distal of the central incisors?

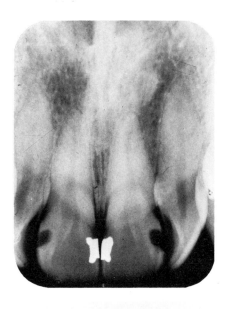

FIGURE 3–2

1. With what metals might this patient's prosthesis be made?

2. With what material are the crowns of the anterior teeth restored?

3. What are the radiopaque lines seen in the cervical area of the anterior teeth?

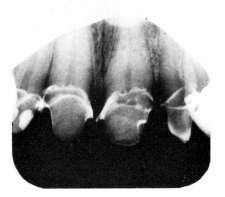

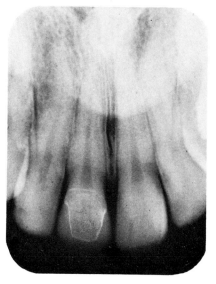

FIGURE 3–3

What type of crown has been placed on the right central incisor?

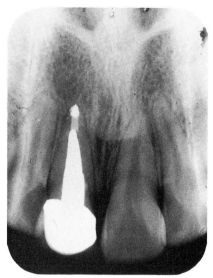

FIGURE 3-4

What restorative materials have been used to treat the right central incisor?

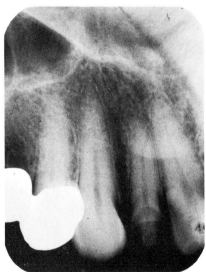

FIGURE 3-5

What material has been used to restore the crown of the lateral incisor?

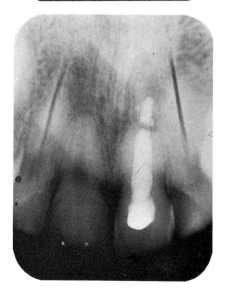

FIGURE 3-6

1. What material has been used to restore the crown of the right central incisor?

2. What might the two radiopaque dots represent?

3. What other materials are seen in this radiograph?

4. What is the cause of the radiolucent lines at the upper corners of this film?

FIGURE 3-7

This 23 year old patient presented for a routine examination. The full-mouth radiographic survey revealed a radiopaque object on the cervical third of the root of the left central incisor. There was no restoration on this tooth, and it was vital. There was no history of pain. With careful questioning, the patient revealed that she had been involved in an automobile accident several months earlier.

1. What is your most likely diagnosis of this radiopacity?

2. What are some other circumstances or objects that might produce a similar radiographic picture?

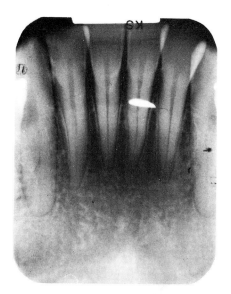

FIGURE 3-8

1. What is the approximate age of this patient? How do you know?

2. Is the right central incisor in lingual or labial version? Give the reason for your answer.

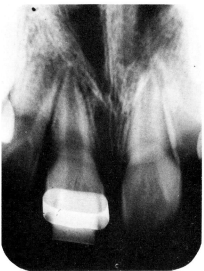

FIGURE 3-9

1. What is the name of the appliance seen in this radiograph?

2. Does this appear to be a young or elderly patient? Give the reason for your answer.

3. What was the probable reason for initiating this type of therapy?

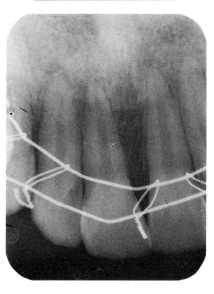

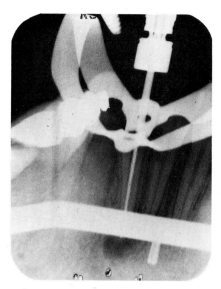

FIGURE 3–10

Name five metallic objects that can be identified in this radiograph.

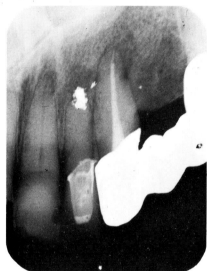

FIGURE 3–11

1. What two forms of endodontic therapy may be seen in this radiograph?

2. Name two reasons why the lateral incisor was not treated in a manner similar to that used to treat the cuspid.

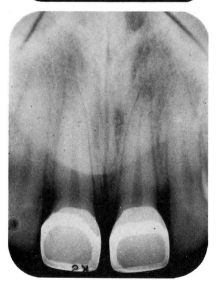

FIGURE 3–12

With what material are the central incisors restored?

Viewing from left to right, tell what materials the arrows are pointing to in each of the following radiographs.

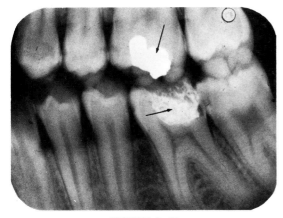

FIGURE 3–13

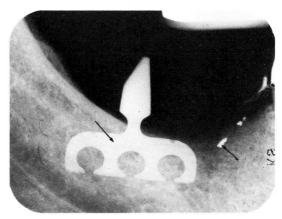

FIGURE 3–14

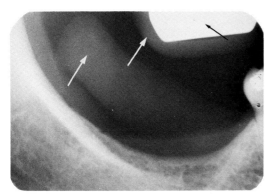

FIGURE 3–15

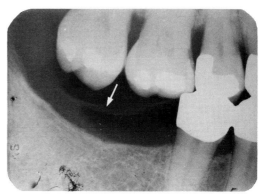

FIGURE 3–16

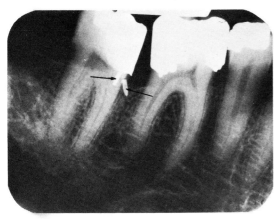

FIGURE 3–17

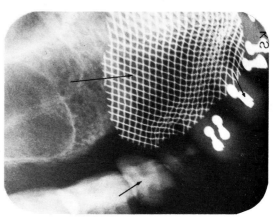

FIGURE 3–18

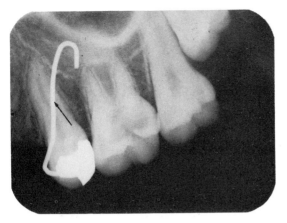

FIGURE 3–19

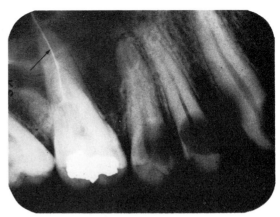

FIGURE 3–20

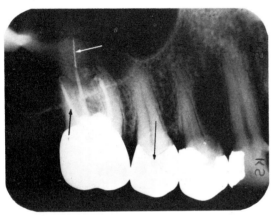

FIGURE 3–21

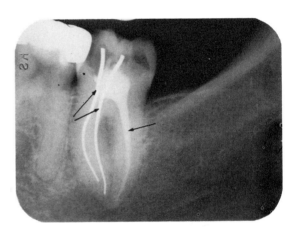

FIGURE 3–22

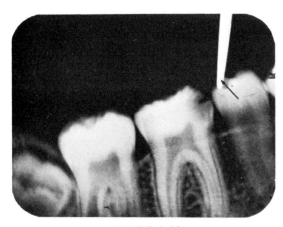

FIGURE 3–23

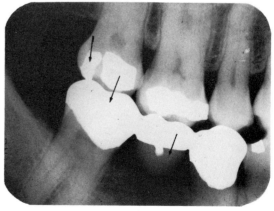

FIGURE 3–24

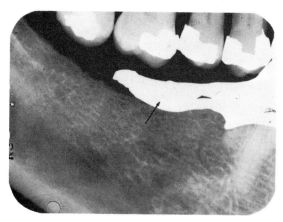

FIGURE 3–25

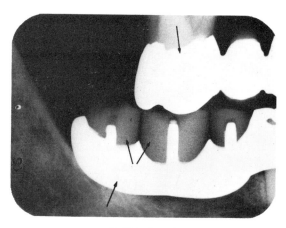

FIGURE 3–26

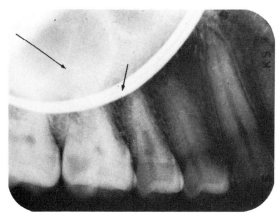

FIGURE 3–27

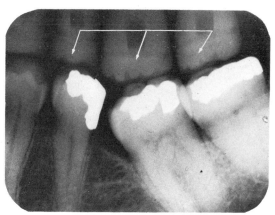

FIGURE 3–28

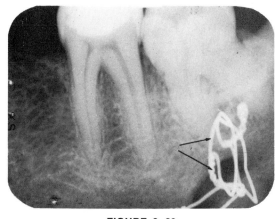

FIGURE 3–29

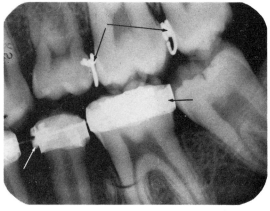

FIGURE 3–30

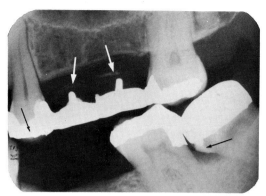

FIGURE 3-31

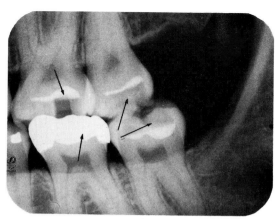

FIGURE 3-32

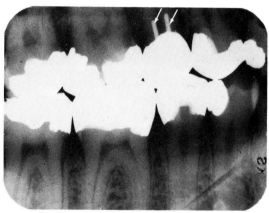

FIGURE 3-33

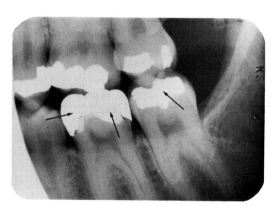

FIGURE 3-34

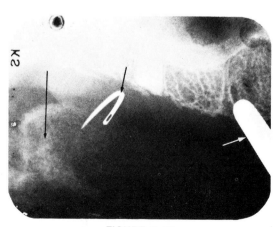

FIGURE 3-35

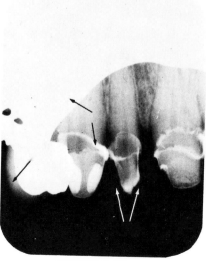

FIGURE 3-36

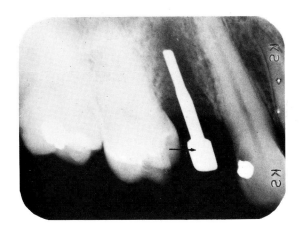

FIGURE 3–37

FIGURE 3–38

What materials were used to restore the mandibular second deciduous molar seen in this radiograph?

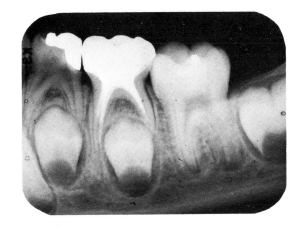

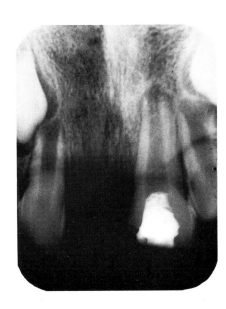

FIGURE 3–39

What material was used in this fractured central incisor?

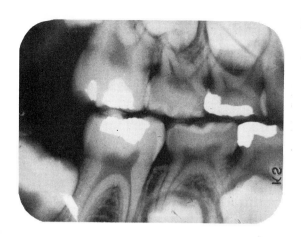

FIGURE 3-40

This young patient was fond of eating baked potatoes. What, do you suppose, is the radiopaque object superimposed on the distal root of the mandibular first permanent molar?

SECTION 4

DEVELOPMENTAL ANOMALIES
AND
PATHOLOGIC ENTITIES

FIGURE 4-1

Mr. John Smith is 37 years old. You're looking at a routine periapical radiograph of a mandibular left molar. The patient said that the area was asymptomatic and that the mandibular left third molar was extracted approximately five years earlier.

1. Is this radiograph suggestive of a benign or a malignant lesion?

2. What is the most likely diagnosis?

3. If there were no previous history of extraction, what would be the most likely diagnosis?

4. How would you obtain a definitive diagnosis?

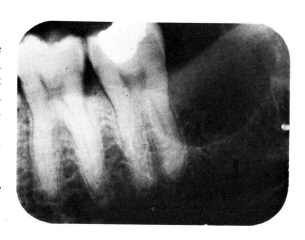

FIGURE 4-2

1. Describe the radiographic appearance of the mandibular first permanent molar seen in this radiograph.

2. What pathologic entities can be seen?

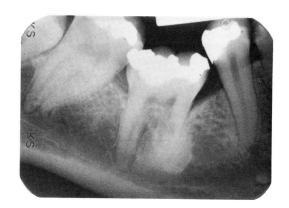

FIGURE 4-3

Marie Danielle, a 13 year old female, plays floor hockey, a popular Canadian school sport. She is asymptomatic. This radiolucency was discovered during a routine dental check-up. Upon questioning, she stated she was struck on the face with a hockey puck and that her jaw was quite sore for a few days.

1. With this history and radiograph, what is the most likely diagnosis?

2. What simple clinical test would be helpful in making a provisional diagnosis?

3. How would you obtain a definitive diagnosis?

4. Name four central lesions of bone that may have a similar radiographic appearance and a tendency to occur in this area.

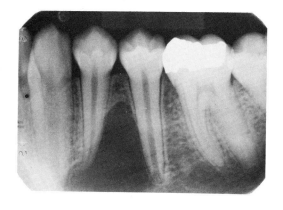

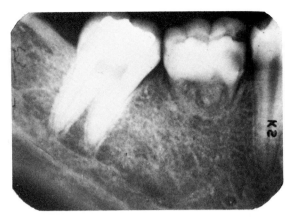

FIGURE 4-4

Mary Sweet, a 24 year old female, was involved as a patient in a dental research project when she was 18. Her nontreatable carious mandibular first permanent molar was extracted as part of the dental treatment.

1. According to the radiograph, what do you suppose that treatment procedure was?

2. Describe the radiographic appearance of the tooth occupying the place of the mandibular first molar.

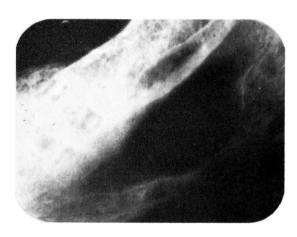

FIGURE 4-5

Sam Graingrower, a 52 year old farmer, presented to his dentist with a complaint of a tingling sensation on the left side of his lower lip. He was edentulous from the mandibular left first premolar posterior. This radiograph shows a view of the mandibular left molar area.

1. Does the lesion appear benign or malignant?

2. What is your differential diagnosis? State pros and cons for each alternative.

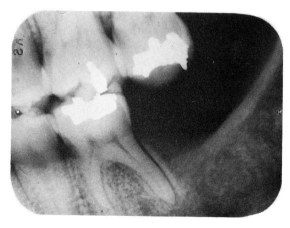

FIGURE 4-6

1. Give a differential diagnosis of a thickened periodontal membrane space.

2. Using this radiograph, substantiate your choice in this particular case. The patient is asymptomatic, and all teeth are vital.

FIGURE 4–7

As the consulting radiologist, what three conditions associated with the mandibular second molar would you note in this radiograph?

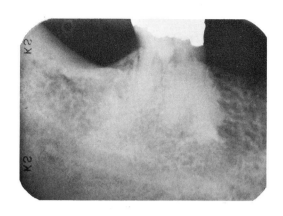

FIGURE 4–8

1. What is the main problem depicted in this radiograph?

2. What notation would you make on the patient's chart concerning the second molar?

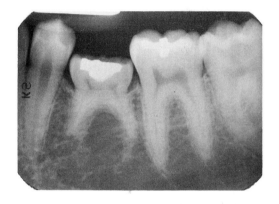

FIGURE 4–9

The features in this radiograph are pathognomonic of what factitial injury to the mandibular second bicuspid?

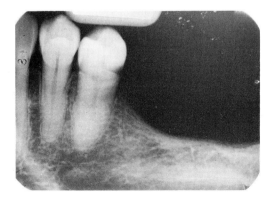

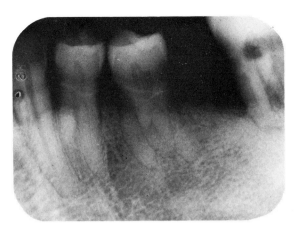

FIGURE 4-10

1. In viewing this radiograph, what abnormalities can you discern regarding the following:
   a. the occlusal surfaces,
   b. pulp chambers,
   c. cervical area, and
   d. roots.

2. Name two other periodontally notable pathologic processes seen in this radiograph.

3. What film-handling error was made in the taking of this radiograph?

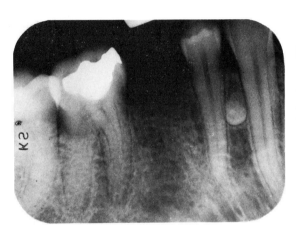

FIGURE 4-11

1. Name the two most likely explanations for the small radiopacity seen between the roots of the cuspid and first bicuspid teeth.

2. Which odontogenic cyst commonly develops in this area?

3. Name four other radiopaque entities commonly seen in this area.

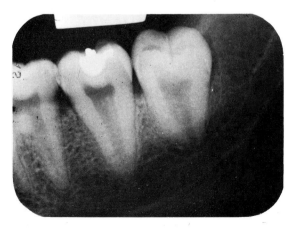

FIGURE 4-12

How would you describe the root shape of the molars in this radiograph?

FIGURE 4-13

1. What term is used to describe the radiographic appearance of the first molar in this radiograph?

2. With what syndromes may this tooth form be associated?

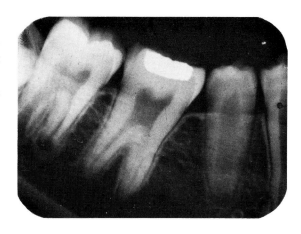

FIGURE 4-14

1. What is the most obvious abnormality seen in this radiograph?

2. Name two conditions with which this abnormality may be associated.

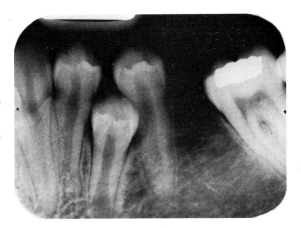

FIGURE 4-15

Cherry Lee is a 13 year old female who has had this problem since age three. Clinically, her face appears swollen bilaterally and is asymptomatic. Radiographically, bilateral multilocular expansile lesions are noted in both the mandible and maxilla, and there are many congenitally missing and malformed permanent teeth.

1. What is your diagnosis?

2. Can this condition be diagnosed from radiographs alone?

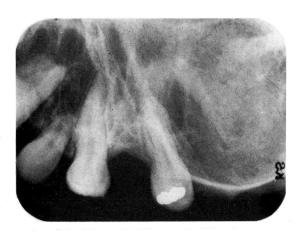

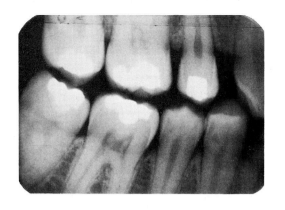

FIGURE 4–16

This bite-wing radiograph was taken during the routine recall examination of John Stone, a 22 year old dental student. He was completely asymptomatic except for the fact that he complained of too much school work.

1. Name three separate radiopaque conditions associated with the pulps of this teeth.

2. Which is the most significant? Why?

3. Which is the least significant?

FIGURE 4–17

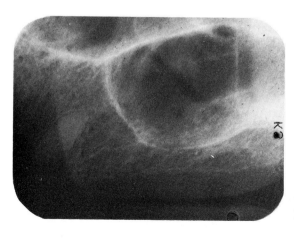

Belinda Brokenbone is a 24 year old female who has had a long history of fractures of the long bones. She is very small in stature and is confined to a wheelchair. Her eyes are blue and so is the sclera. Clinically, her teeth appear to have normal shape and size. She has a low caries history. When she smiles, as she often does, her anterior teeth appear to have an opalescent sheen.

1. What is Belinda's systemic condition?

2. What developmental dental defect is involved?

3. What features of this condition are seen radiographically?

FIGURE 4–18

1. In viewing this radiograph, what finding would you report?

2. a. Where is it located?

b. What prominent radiographic landmark helps you with this location?

3. Which anatomic structure produced the well-delineated vertical line near the left edge of the radiograph?

FIGURE 4-19

1. Give your differential diagnosis of the condition represented by the radiopacity at the inferior border of the mandible.

2. How would you proceed radiographically in order to obtain a more definitive diagnosis?

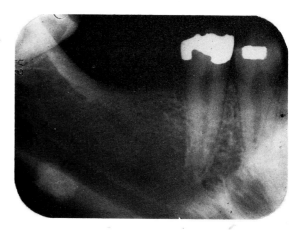

FIGURE 4-20

This is a periapical radiograph taken as part of the routine full-mouth radiographic survey of a 46 year old black edentulous female. She is currently asymptomatic.

1. Which anatomic area is shown on this radiograph?

2. Give a differential diagnosis of the lesions seen.

3. Which alternative is your most likely choice?

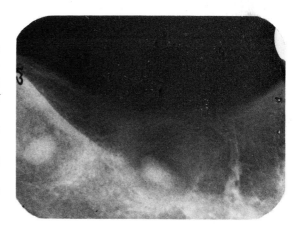

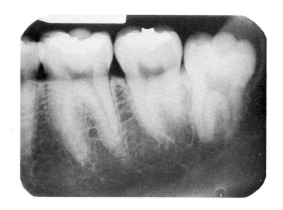

FIGURE 4-21

1. What condition is present in the roots of the mandibular second molar?

2. What was the probable cause of this condition?

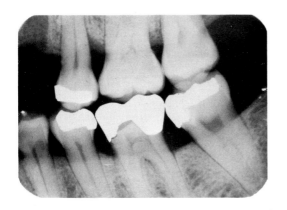

FIGURE 4–22

1. What does the radiolucent area beneath the restoration in the mandibular first molar represent?

2. What does the radiopaque area beneath the restoration in the mandibular second molar represent?

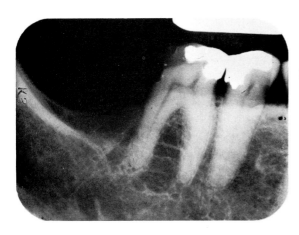

FIGURE 4–23

Comment on the trabecular pattern of the alveolar bone between the roots of the mandibular first molar.

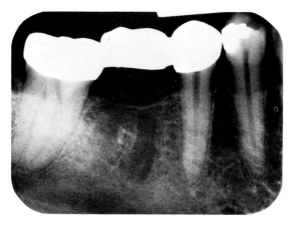

FIGURE 4–24

The three-unit bridge seen in this radiograph was constructed shortly after the first molar was extracted. The patient has been wearing the bridge for seven years, yet the alveolar pattern beneath the pontic does not appear normal.

1. From the radiograph, what is your diagnosis?

2. How would you confirm this?

FIGURE 4-25

1. Give a differential diagnosis of the radiopaque lesion seen in the maxillary antrum.

2. What is the most likely choice?

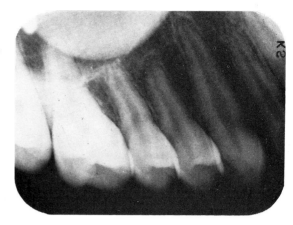

FIGURE 4-26

What unusual entity do you see in this radiograph?

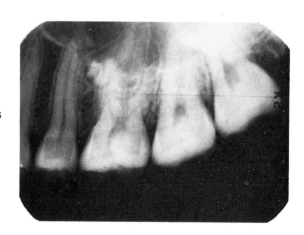

FIGURE 4-27

This 19 year old patient presented to the office with swelling of the right side of his face, low-grade fever, earache, and trismus. The radiograph was difficult to take owing to the trismus and some sensitivity in the molar area.

1. What is your diagnosis?

2. Will the third molar erupt any further? Give the reason for your answer.

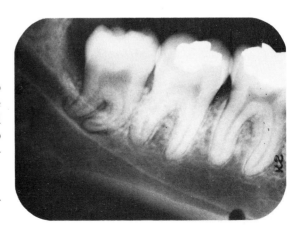

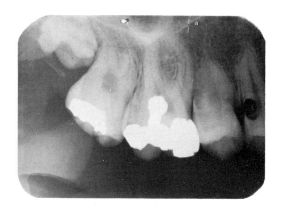

FIGURE 4-28

This 17 year old female had Hodgkin's disease at age nine. The only manifestations of the disease were low-grade fever and cervical lymphadenopathy that persisted even after three weeks of antibiotic treatment. She received the usual mode of therapy and is presently free of disease.

1. What is the common mode of therapy?
2. What effect did this have on her teeth?

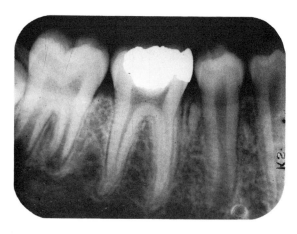

FIGURE 4-29

1. How old is this patient?
2. What pathologic entity is present?

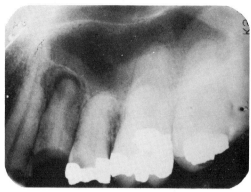

A

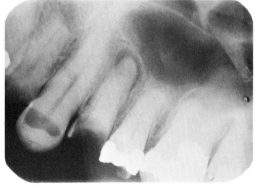

B

FIGURE 4–30

In radiograph *A*, our patient has a completely carious first bicuspid with chronic periapical disease. Radiograph *B* was taken one week after radiograph *A*, during which time potassium penicillin G had been taken t.i.d., with a total daily dose of 3,000,000 international units.

1. What is your differential diagnosis of the pathologic condition associated with the apex of the first bicuspid? (Be thorough.)

2. What effect has the antibiotic therapy had on these periapical tissues?

FIGURE 4–31

1. Compare the radiographic appearance of the pulps of the mandibular second bicuspid and the first molar.

2. How would you treat these pulps? Give your reasons for this treatment.

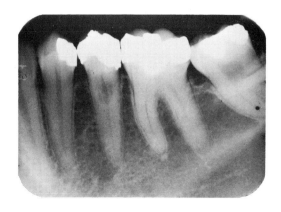

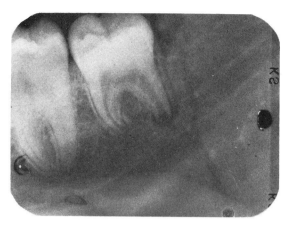

FIGURE 4-32

George Lovejoy is a 19 year old college student who attended his older sister's wedding reception two days before his problem began. Thanks to a copious flow of pink champagne, George was feeling no pain but vaguely remembers hitting himself in the face with the refrigerator door in response to an urgent request for more ice cubes. His chief complaint was that his jaw "hurt" when he masticated food. The third molar was vital.

What is your diagnosis?

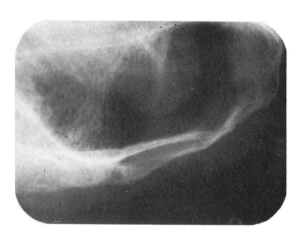

FIGURE 4-33

What lesion is present in the maxillary sinus?

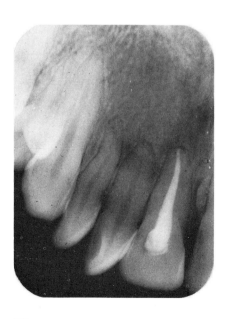

FIGURE 4-34

What developmental anomaly can be clearly seen in this radiograph?

FIGURE 4–35

What developmental defects can you detect in this periapical radiograph of an eight year old boy?

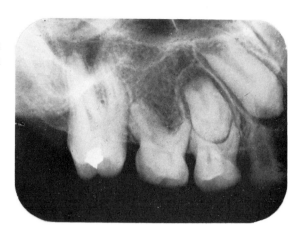

FIGURE 4–36

1. Where is this radiopacity located?
2. What does it represent?
3. What alterations have occurred in association with this radiopacity?
4. How would you treat this?

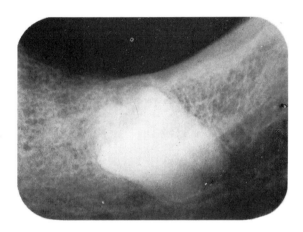

FIGURE 4–37

1. In what area of the mouth was this radiograph taken?
2. What pathologic process do you observe?
3. What tooth (teeth) previously occupied this area? State the reason for your answer.
4. Was this tooth extracted recently?
5. From this radiograph, what type of soft-tissue ridge would you expect to find clinically?

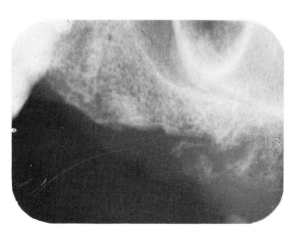

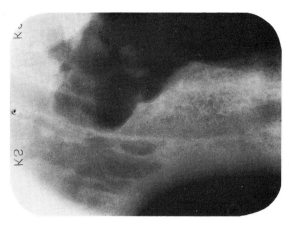

FIGURE 4-38

This is a radiograph of a 39 year old male patient taken one week after surgery. Because the surgery was performed in a foreign country, the pathology report was not available. The patient stated that the lesion was found to be benign and that he had been unaware of its presence. The surgeon had recommended periodic check-ups of the area.

1. What was the location and extent of the lesion?

2. What appears to have been the mode of therapy?

3. Which two odontogenic lesions would you strongly suspect?

4. Would you reevaluate and follow this case closely? State the reasons for your answer.

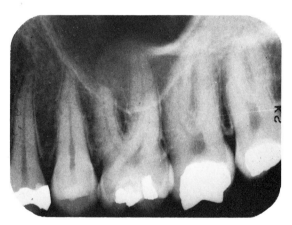

FIGURE 4-39

What radiopaque lesion may be seen in the maxillary sinus? (You've seen this before.)

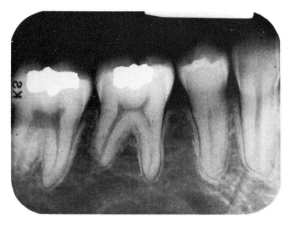

FIGURE 4-40

1. Identify the following radiolucencies:

    a. the crest of the ridge between the second bicuspid and the first molar and

    b. the one near the apex of the second bicuspid.

2. What iatrogenic dentistry was done here?

3. What other pathologic dental finding is evident?

FIGURE 4-41

What entity do the two radiolucencies at the crest of the ridge represent?

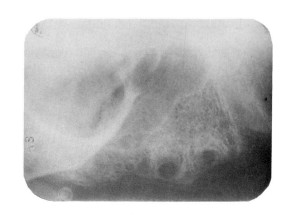

FIGURE 4-42

1. What developmental anomaly do you see here?

2. What structure do the two thin radiopaque lines at the apex of the mesial root of the mandibular first molar represent?

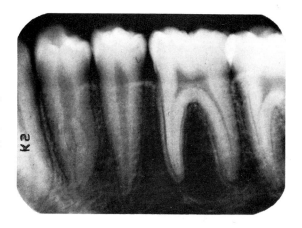

FIGURE 4-43

This 24 year old male patient presented with a severe pain in the mandible that he could not localize to one particular tooth. Until now he has been able to control the pain with aspirin.

1. What questions would you ask the patient?

2. What objective tests would you perform?

3. Using this radiograph, give a differential diagnosis.

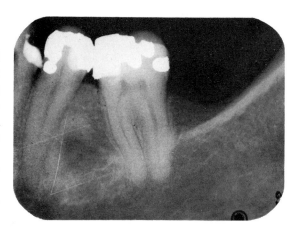

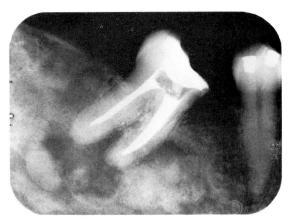

FIGURE 4-44

This 57 year old male patient has a history of pain in the weight-bearing joints. The alkaline phosphatase level is 156 Bodansky units. He has had several complete maxillary dentures constructed, each one becoming too tight after several years' use.

1. With the aid of the radiograph, tell what condition this history suggests.

2. What radiographic features of this condition can be seen here?

3. What other condition does this radiograph closely resemble?

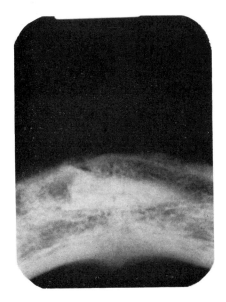

FIGURE 4-45

In reviewing this radiograph, what points of interest should you note?

FIGURE 4-46

Describe and locate the entity represented by the central radiopacity in this radiograph.

FIGURE 4–47

1. What developmental anomaly is seen here?

2. Would you suspect that this radiopacity is located more palatally or labially?

3. How else could you locate this structure?

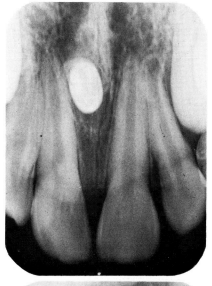

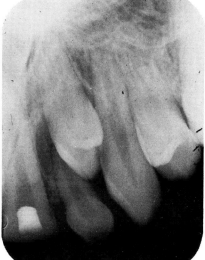

FIGURE 4–48

What term is used to describe this particular set of circumstances?

FIGURE 4–49

1. What term is used to describe the clinical appearance of the coronal portion of the lateral incisor?

2. What other anomaly can be seen?

3. What treatment would you recommend?

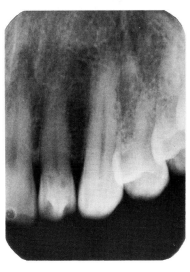

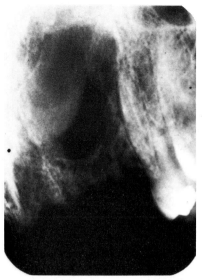

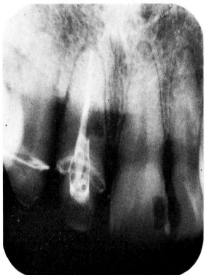

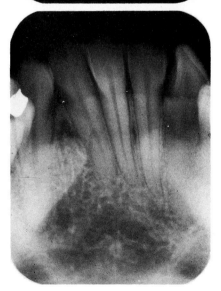

FIGURE 4-50

1. What normal anatomic structure appears to be superimposed upon this radiolucent lesion?

2. What is your differential diagnosis of this lesion?

FIGURE 4-51

1. What pathologic condition is notable in this radiograph?

2. What type of restoration was used for the lateral incisor and cuspid?

FIGURE 4-52

1. Toward what endodontically significant structure does the radiopacity on the left of the radiograph appear to be pointing?

2. What are these bilateral radiopaque structures?

FIGURE 4-53

What would you interpret the multiple radiopacities seen in the central portion of this radiograph to represent?

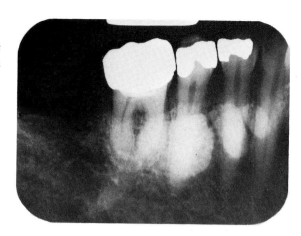

FIGURE 4-54

What would you interpret the bilateral radiopaque structures seen in the lower corners of this radiograph to represent?

After checking your answers, take a break.

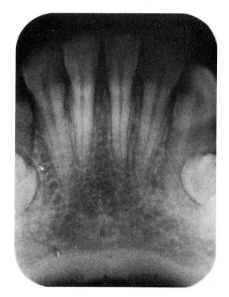

Welcome back. Ready to start again? Here we go.

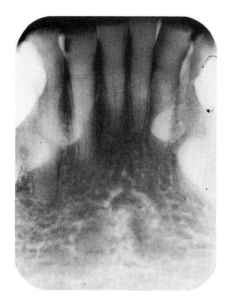

FIGURE 4-55

Name at least five separate findings that you should report from your observation of this radiograph.

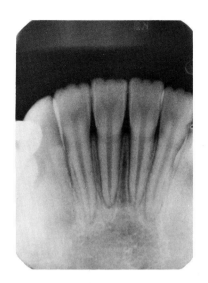

FIGURE 4–56

What term is used to describe the notched appearance of the mandibular incisor teeth?

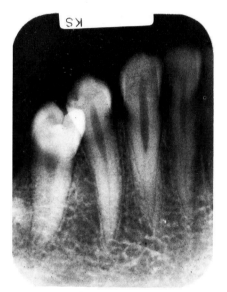

FIGURE 4–57

What developmental anomaly can be seen in this radiograph?

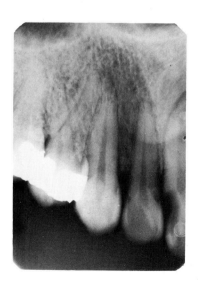

FIGURE 4–58

Identify the following radiopacities:

1. the teardrop-shaped radiopacity near the bifurcation area of the maxillary first bicuspid,

2. the oval-shaped radiopacity in the coronal area of the maxillary cuspid,

3. the crescent-shaped radiopacity associated with the apices of the maxillary lateral and central incisors, and

4. the curved, horizontal radiopaque line on the cervical third of the root of the maxillary lateral incisor.

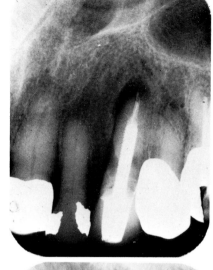

FIGURE 4-59

1. In viewing this radiograph, what notations would you make concerning the maxillary cuspid?

2. With what type of restoration was this tooth restored?

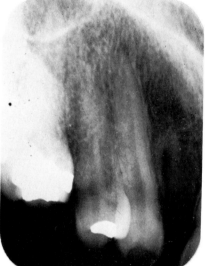

FIGURE 4-60

What is your impression of the vertical radiolucency mesial to the maxillary cuspid?

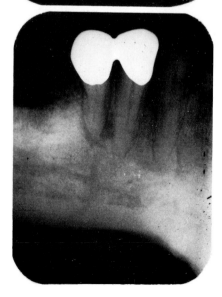

FIGURE 4-61

This 48 year old male patient has been visiting his physician off and on for over a year. Antibiotics were prescribed that would help for a short time, but a lesion on his skin kept recurring. The physician did not suspect the teeth because there was no toothache and the teeth appeared sound.

1. What is your diagnosis?

2. What treatment would you recommend?

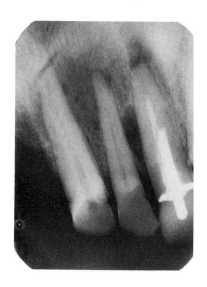

FIGURE 4-62

1. You are a very astute radiologist and have been given this rather poor film to interpret. The patient has an acute toothache in the maxillary right anterior area. Which tooth is the culprit?

2. Note the cluster of nutrient foramina between the lateral incisor and cuspid teeth. What central lesion of bone may be associated with these?

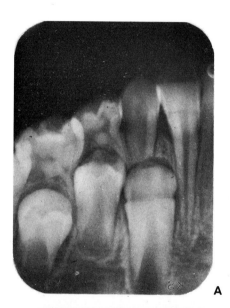

A

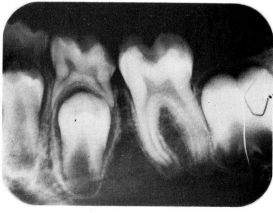

B

FIGURE 4-63

These two radiographs are from the same patient.

1. How old is the patient?

2. What developmental defect is present?

3. What teeth are affected?

FIGURE 4–64

1. What does the radiopaque line in the cervical area of the central, lateral, and cuspid teeth represent?

2. What technical error was made on this radiograph?

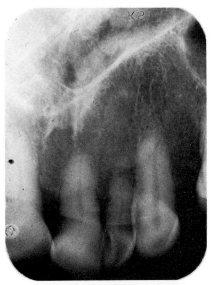

FIGURE 4–65

How would you account for the radiopaque semicircular area seen in the lower portion of this radiograph? Be careful!

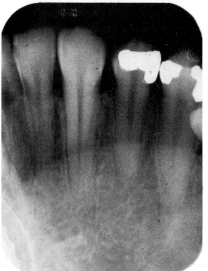

FIGURE 4–66

What developmental defect may be visualized here? Let's see how good you are.

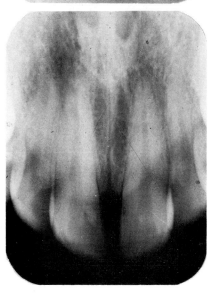

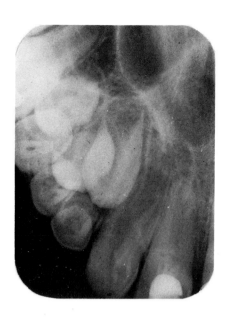

FIGURE 4-67

1. What developmental defect is seen here?

2. How old is this patient?

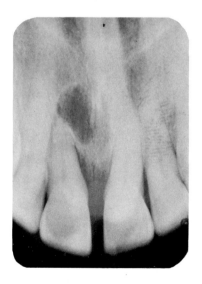

FIGURE 4-68

1. Which developmental cyst occurs in this area?

2. Which other developmental cyst also occurs in this area but is not central in bone?

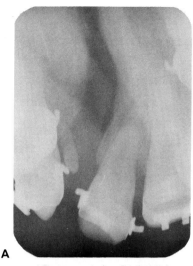

A

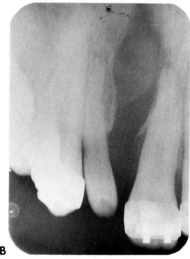

B

FIGURE 4–69

1. What developmental defect of the jaws do you see?

2. What other developmental defect is present?

3. What structure does the oval-shaped radiopacity in the middle of the defect represent?

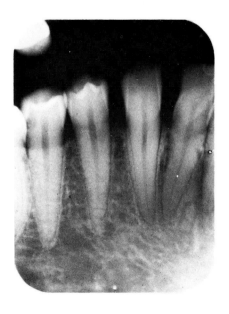

FIGURE 4–70

What term is used to describe the spaces between these teeth?

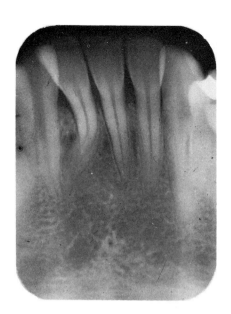

FIGURE 4-71

What term is used to describe the malformation seen in this radiograph?

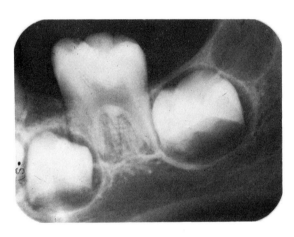

FIGURE 4-72

This patient is seven years old. What is your radiographic impression of the radiolucency just distal to the last molar?

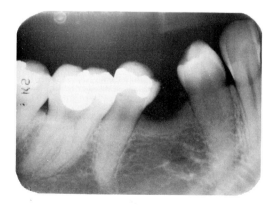

FIGURE 4-73

The only tooth that this patient has ever lost is the right mandibular permanent first molar. What term is used to describe the phenomenon that has occurred here?

FIGURE 4-74

This patient is now 11 years old. He had high fevers when he was very young.

1. Estimate within one year the age at which the fever probably occurred.

2. What was the result of this fever?

3. What other teeth, not shown here, could have been affected?

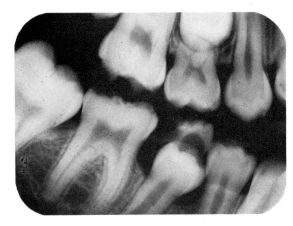

FIGURE 4-75

This 10 year old patient just had a recall examination. Although he has no caries in his permanent dentition, he has a history of having an abscessed first deciduous molar, which has just exfoliated.

After viewing this radiograph, what would you report?

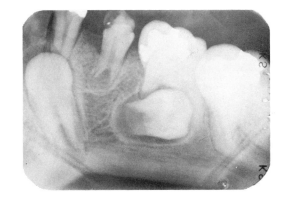

FIGURE 4-76

Johnny Every is 21 years old and is having slight discomfort in the posterior portion of his mouth. Upon examination, you notice that the gingiva on the crest of the ridge distal to the second molar appears swollen and slightly bluish in color. This radiograph was taken at the time of examination. No treatment was given. The patient was asymptomatic within 15 days.

What is your diagnosis?

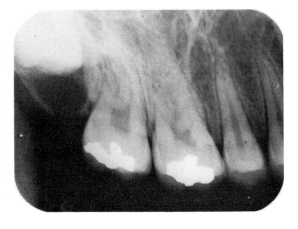

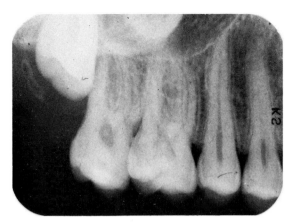

FIGURE 4-77

What is your diagnosis of the small radiopacity associated with the crown of the erupting third molar?

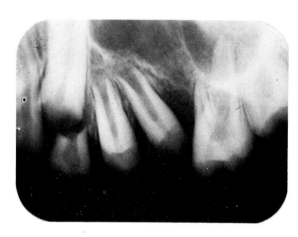

FIGURE 4-78

The features depicted in this radiograph are pathognomonic of what condition?

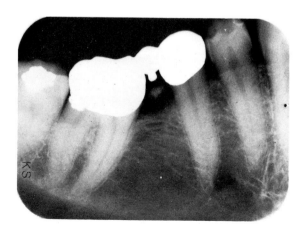

FIGURE 4-79

What is your impression of
1. the pontic material,
2. the radiopacity associated with the pontic, and
3. the radiolucency at the apex of the second bicuspid.

FIGURE 4-80

1. What is your impression of the radio-pacity associated with the mesial root of the mandibular first molar?

2. Is this the common location for this lesion?

3. What is the treatment? Give the reasons for your answer.

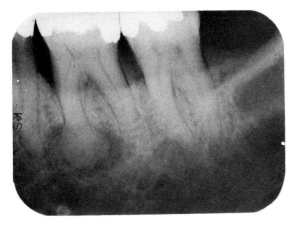

FIGURE 4-81

1. What radiolucent lesion(s) is(are) present that may lead to tooth loss?

2. What radiopaque entity is present and may lead to alveolar bone loss?

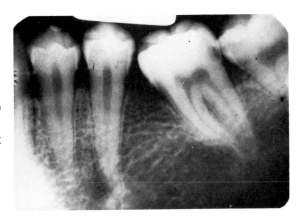

FIGURE 4-82

1. What radiopaque entity is present that may lead to alveolar bone loss?

2. Of the three teeth seen in this radiograph, which one do you suppose would be the most difficult to extract?

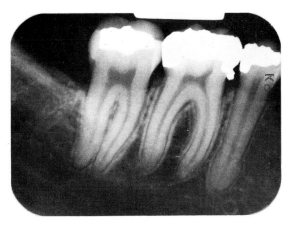

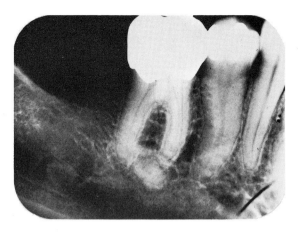

FIGURE 4–83

This radiograph was part of a routine full-mouth survey of a 43 year old black female. Preparing a small hole in the occlusal of the crown without the aid of anesthesia revealed that the mandibular first molar was vital. The patient was asymptomatic.

What is your impression of the following two radiopacities associated with the mandibular first molar:

1. the radiopacity at the apex of the mesial root, and

2. the radiopacity in the bifurcation area.

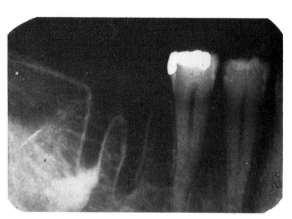

FIGURE 4–84

With the help of this radiograph, explain the reason for the extraction of the mandibular first molar.

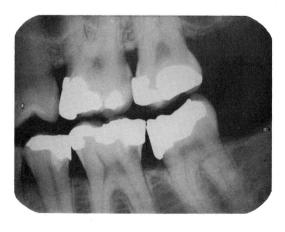

FIGURE 4–85

Name the conditions present in the following locations:

1. the distal of the maxillary second bicuspid,

2. the distal of the maxillary first molar,

3. the distal of the mandibular second bicuspid,

4. the distal of the mandibular first molar, and

5. the mesial of the mandibular second molar.

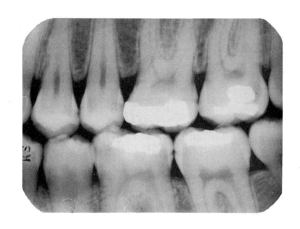

FIGURE 4-86

Locate all carious lesions and indicate whether they are incipient (decalcification) or frank caries.

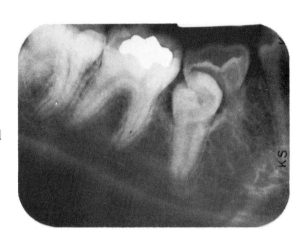

FIGURE 4-87

Will the mandibular second bicuspid erupt?

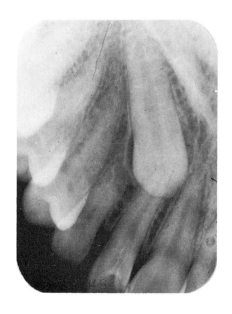

FIGURE 4-88

After viewing this radiograph, what do you report? Be thorough.

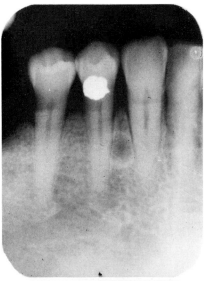

FIGURE 4-89

1. What is the probable cause of the horizontal line on the cervical third of the roots of the mandibular second bicuspid and cuspid?

2. What is the most likely diagnosis of the radiolucency between the mandibular cuspid and first bicuspid teeth?

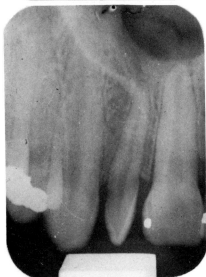

FIGURE 4-90

How would you describe the shape of the maxillary lateral incisor?

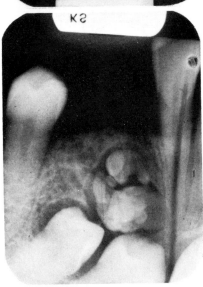

FIGURE 4-91

1. What is your interpretation of the odontogenic pathologic condition seen on this radiograph?

2. Would you send the surgical specimen in for biopsy? Give the reasons for your answer.

FIGURE 4–92

1. What anatomic structure do the radiolucent vertical lines represent?

2. What is the radiopaque material in the cervical area of these teeth?

3. With what disease may the preceding entities be associated?

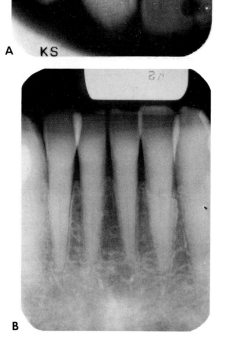

A   KS

B

FIGURE 4–93

1. What pulpal condition do these two radiographs demonstrate?

2. What is the significance of this in case *A*?

3. What is the significance of this in case *B*?

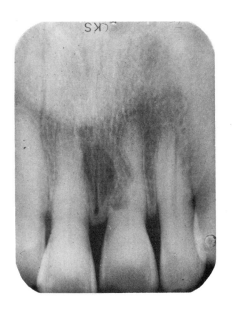

FIGURE 4-94

1. What common developmental cyst occurs in this area?

2. What uncommon finding is seen here?

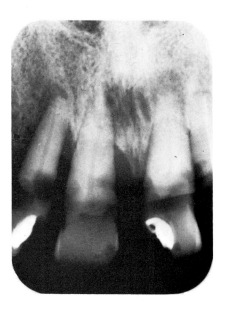

FIGURE 4-95

Beginning with those at the apices and working toward those at the incisal aspects, list the common conditions that can be seen radiographically in association with all three of these teeth. Give a differential diagnosis where possible.

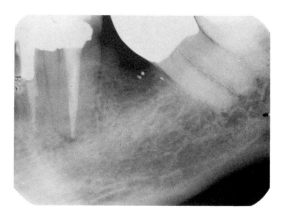

FIGURE 4-96

1. The three radiopaque spots seen in the bone near the crest of the ridge in this radiograph are most likely _____

_____.

2. Clinically, a smooth, firm nodule was palpable on the buccal aspect of the crest of the ridge. This is most likely ___

_____.

FIGURE 4-97

1. What term is used to describe the relationship of these maxillary molars to the mandibular ridge?
2. Name the two contributing causes.

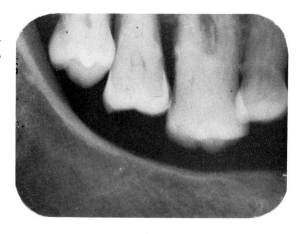

FIGURE 4-98

1. Describe the appearance of the alveolar bone in this radiograph.
2. What is the differential diagnosis?

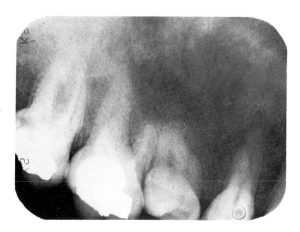

FIGURE 4-99

Give a differential diagnosis of the radiopaque material seen in this radiograph.

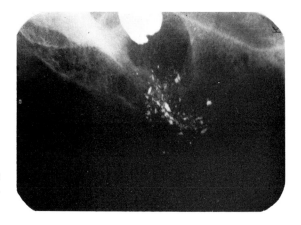

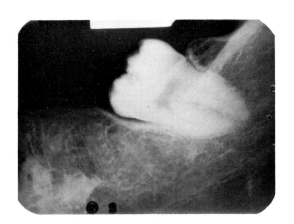

FIGURE 4-100

What anatomic variation can be seen in this radiograph?

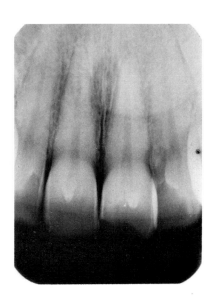

FIGURE 4-101

1. What anatomic structure produces the semicircular radiopacity at the apical third of the root of the left central incisor?

2. What anatomic structure produces the radiopaque line along the incisal third of these anterior teeth?

3. Why may one or more of these teeth be nonvital?

4. a. What developmental anomaly can be seen in association with the crowns of the central incisor?

    b. What analogous condition may be seen on the occlusal of the mandibular bicuspid teeth of Oriental persons?

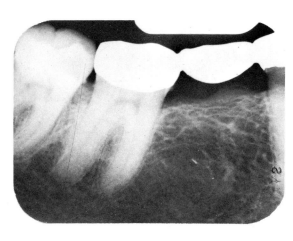

FIGURE 4-102

What term is used to describe the radiopaque bump on the alveolar ridge under the pontic?

FIGURE 4-103

In the event of caries, would the bicuspid teeth seen in this radiograph be more susceptibile to an early pulpitis than normally? Give the reason for your answer.

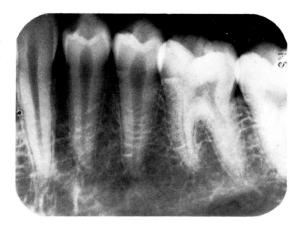

FIGURE 4-104

Name two developmental anomalies that can be seen to be developing in this radiograph.

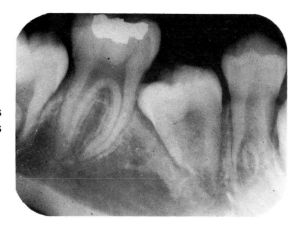

FIGURE 4-105

Relative to the size of the teeth seen in this radiograph, what term is used to describe this developmental condition?

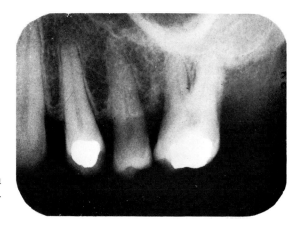

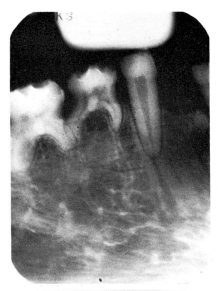

FIGURE 4–106

1. What pathologic entities can be seen in this radiograph?

2. What condition is compatible with the pathologic findings in this radiograph?

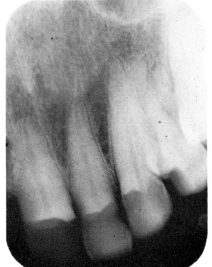

FIGURE 4–107

What change can be seen in the crowns of these teeth?

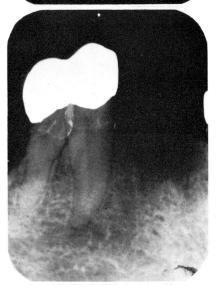

FIGURE 4–108

What material is visualized as a radiopaque line in the cervical portion of these teeth?

FIGURE 4-109

These three patients have the same condition:

1. What is the probable race of these patients?

2. What is their probable age?

3. What is their probable sex?

4. Are these teeth probably vital?

5. What is the name of their condition?

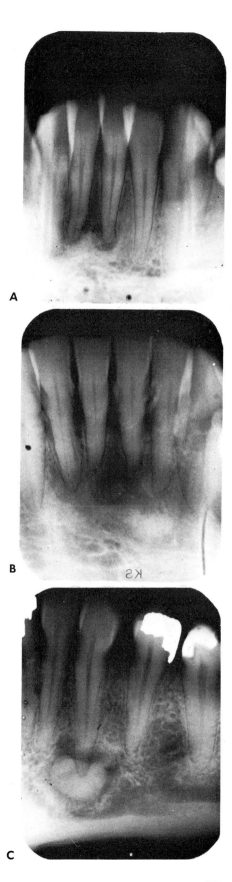

A

B

C

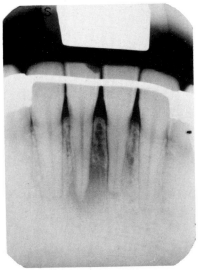

FIGURE 4-110

Both of these central incisors were subject to the same single traumatic blow. Compare the manners in which these two teeth have reacted, their probable vitality, and the modes of treatment required.

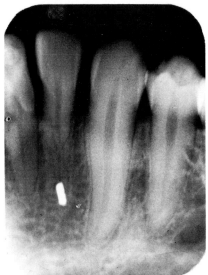

FIGURE 4-111

1. Do you think this patient has a previous history of trauma to his mandibular incisor teeth?

2. What treatment is evident in this radiograph?

3. What would you interpret this radiograph to represent?

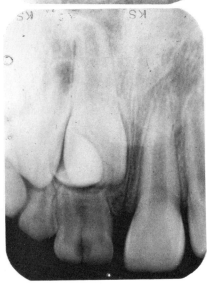

FIGURE 4-112

1. What developmental defect can be seen in association with the right deciduous central and lateral incisors?

2. What is the cause of the delayed eruption of the right permanent central and lateral incisors?

FIGURE 4–113

1. State two theories concerning the etiology of the lateral periodontal cyst seen in this radiograph.

2. Is it possible for this cyst to have a high recurrence rate postoperatively?

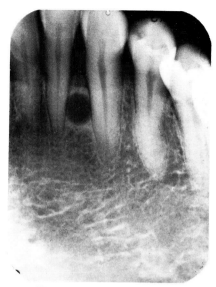

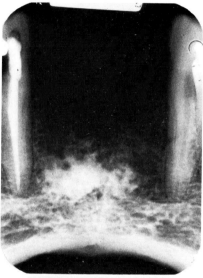

FIGURE 4–114

Name the four radiopacities seen in this radiograph.

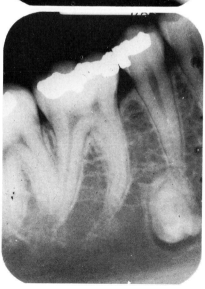

FIGURE 4–115

1. What is your diagnosis of this radiopaque lesion?

2. Are the radiographic findings sufficient to warrant surgical excision?

3. Is the radiographic picture sufficient for use in establishing the final diagnosis of the case? Give the reasons for your answer.

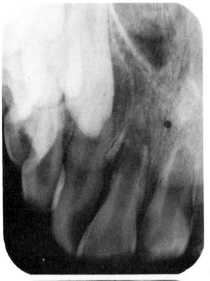

A

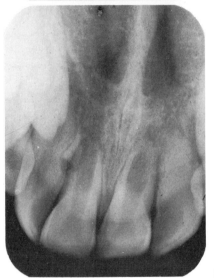

B

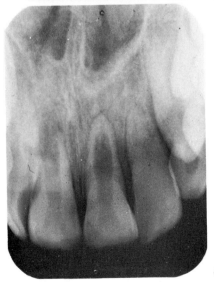

C

FIGURE 4–116

Mary Quitecontrary is a 10 year old female who fell off her bicycle three years ago. Her teeth were sensitive and ached for a short time but eventually felt better. Recently, she has had some mild discomfort in the soft tissue high above the front teeth. Upon examination two parulis were noted in the area of the mucobuccal fold adjacent to the maxillary centrals.

What sequelae of the fall can be noted from these radiographs? Be thorough.

FIGURE 4–117

Jenny Jeans had her mandibular left second premolar extracted several years ago because of a toothache. During a recent dental visit a class II amalgam was placed in the mandibular left first molar. After her visit, she had sensitivity to hot and cold, and eventually a constant toothache developed. Upon reexamination it was found that the first molar was tender to percussion, and this radiograph was taken.

1. What is your diagnosis?
2. Why did this patient have pain?
3. How old is this patient?
4. What developmental anomaly is associated with the aching tooth?

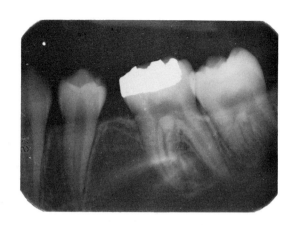

FIGURE 4–118

Identify the physiologic process that has caused these teeth to have this occlusal configuration.

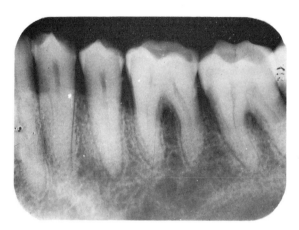

FIGURE 4–119

This 19 year old black female had absolutely perfect dentition upon visual inspection. The soft tissue appeared normal, and the patient was asymptomatic. The routine radiographs showed almost identical lesions in all four quadrants. The oral hygiene was adequate.

What is the most likely diagnosis?

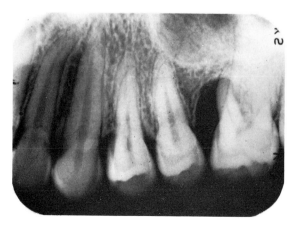

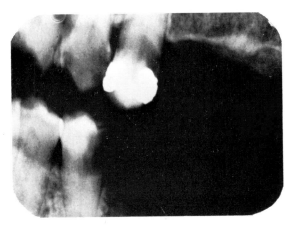

FIGURE 4–120

Mrs. X is a 35 year old female who was treated with cobalt 60 for an oral malignancy.

1. What pathologic process is affecting these teeth?

2. Which tooth shows the most typical lesion?

3. Why do these lesions occur?

4. How can this sequela be prevented?

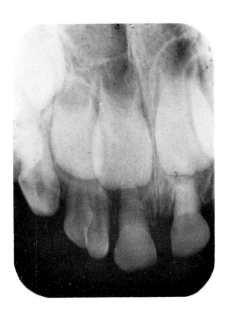

FIGURE 4–121

What developmental anomaly do you see here? Define it.

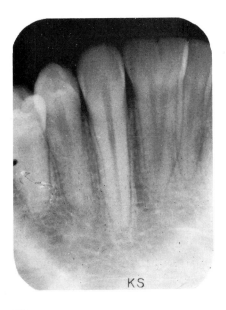

FIGURE 4–122

What developmental anomaly do you see here? Define it. (The tooth on the extreme right of the radiograph is the right central incisor.)

90

FIGURE 4–123

1. What condition is present here?
2. With what fibro-osseous lesion may this be associated?
3. Name two other conditions in which you may find this lesion.

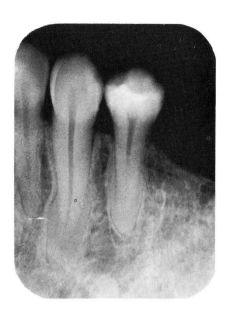

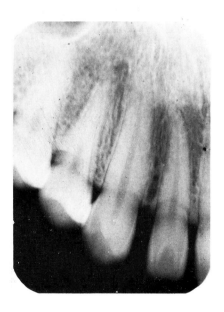

FIGURE 4–124

Look carefully at the cervical area of the lateral incisor. Note the two horizontal lines in this area. What is the cause of these lines?

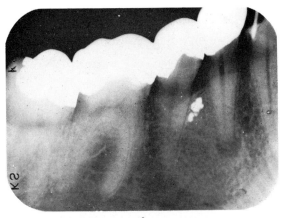

A

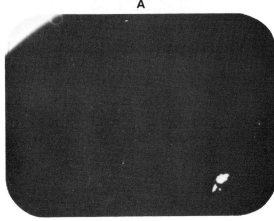

B

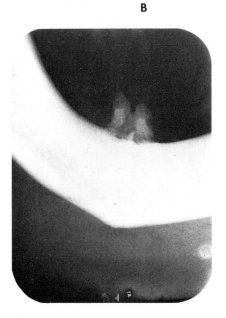

FIGURE 4–125

This 27 year old female patient was no stranger to dental treatment. When the radiopacity between the two bicuspids was noted, the area was checked clinically for the presence of an amalgam tattoo on the alveolar mucosa. No such lesion was seen. Where do you suppose the amalgam tattoo was finally located?

FIGURE 4–126

1. What anatomic variation is seen here?

2. Is this of any clinical significance?

FIGURE 4-127

Give a differential diagnosis for this lesion seen between the central and lateral incisors in a 16 year old black female.

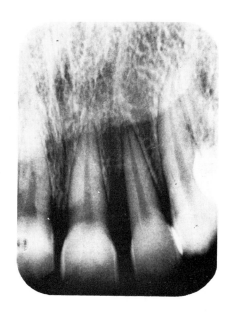

FIGURE 4-128

This patient has a history of an apicoectomy of the maxillary lateral incisor. What condition does the radiolucency in this radiograph represent?

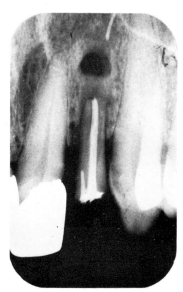

FIGURE 4-129

Would you give this patient a clean bill of health? Give the reasons for your answer.

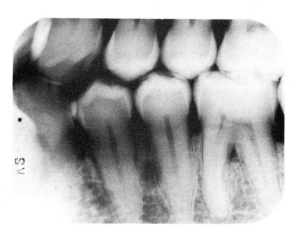

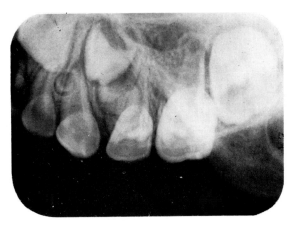

FIGURE 4-130

1. What is the approximate age of this patient?

2. Name the unerupted teeth in this radiograph.

3. Name the undeveloped tooth in this radiograph.

4. Name the radiopaque structure in the lower right-hand corner of the radiograph.

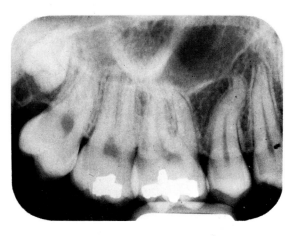

FIGURE 4-131

In viewing this radiograph, what three findings do you note? This 22 year old patient was completely asymptomatic at the time of examination. He has a previous history of chronic sinusitis.

FIGURE 4-132

This 26 year old white female presented with pain in the left mandible and a history of recent weight loss. Further study revealed that after routine extraction of the mandibular left third molar, pain developed. This was unsuccessfully treated for a six-week period with various local dressings in the extraction socket. The patient's husband stated that she had lost 15 pounds and that he frankly suspected that she may have cancer.

Upon examination, several tender lymph nodes were palpable in the left submaxillary area. The extraction socket appeared to contain no clot or granulation tissue. The mandibular left first and second bicuspids were extremely mobile and tested nonvital with the electric pulp test. A fistulous tract could be traced from the lingual of the first molar to an area between the apices of the first and second bicuspids. Radiographically, the trabecular pattern had markedly changed from the normal pattern seen one year earlier. (Fig. A.)

Pulp biopsies of the mandibular first and second bicuspids revealed normal viable pulps. A high-protein diet and antibiotics were prescribed. The patient gradually improved, and penicillin treatment was discontinued after six weeks. Endodontic therapy was completed on the mandibular first and second bicuspids.

What's your diagnosis?

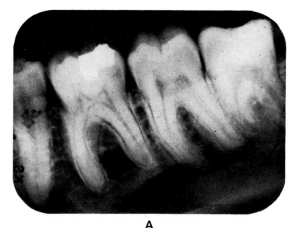

A

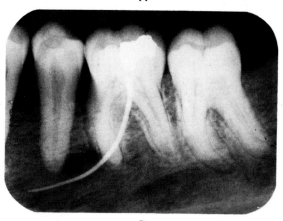

B

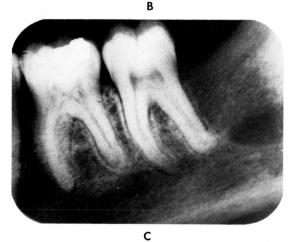

C

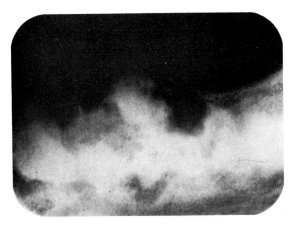

FIGURE 4-133

This 48 year old fully edentulous black female has multiple radiopaque masses throughout the mandible and maxilla. She is asymptomatic and was not aware of here condition.

1. What is her condition?
2. What treatment would you prescribe?

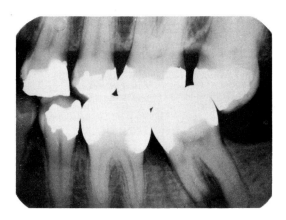

FIGURE 4-134

In looking at this routine bite-wing radiograph, what comments would you make concerning this patient's treatment plan?

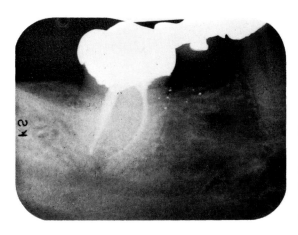

FIGURE 4-135

1. Name two good reasons why endodontics was performed on this molar instead of extraction.
2. What do the little radiopaque specks at the mesial of the molar represent?

FIGURE 4–136

What developing anomaly may be seen in this radiograph?

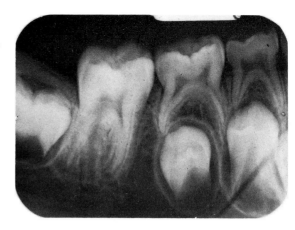

FIGURE 4–137

A biopsy of this asymptomatic lesion on the crest of the mandibular edentulous ridge revealed normal lamellar bone. What is your diagnosis and treatment?

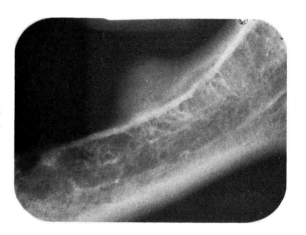

FIGURE 4–138

This routine periapical view revealed a resorbed distal root tip of the mandibular first molar. The patient never had orthodontic treatment or surgery in the area. What is your diagnosis?

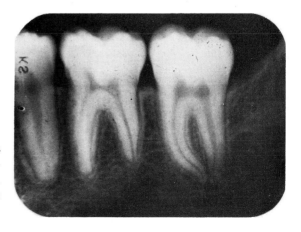

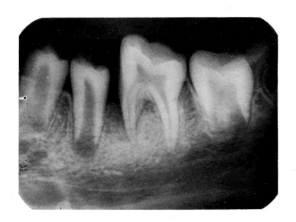

FIGURE 4-139

The features depicted in this radiograph are pathognomonic of what condition? You should know this because you've seen it before.

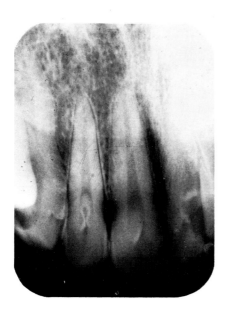

FIGURE 4-140

1. What developmental defect does this radiograph illustrate? (You've seen this before, too.)

2. Unless prevented, what is a frequent sequela?

3. How may this be prevented?

4. What tooth is most commonly affected?

5. Can this defect occur bilaterally?

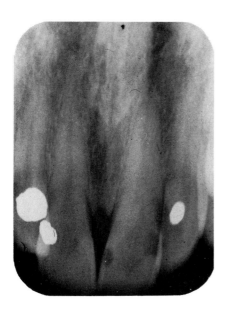

FIGURE 4-141

What developmental defect is illustrated here?

FIGURE 4-142

This should be familiar to you:

1. For what condition does this radiograph present pathognomonic evidence?

2. With what other condition is it sometimes associated?

3. Is this condition hereditary?

4. Are the caries a usual finding?

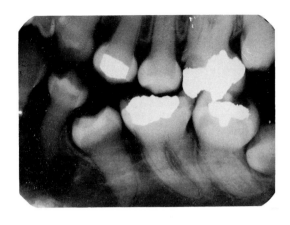

FIGURE 4-143

A 12 year old male presented to the clinic complaining of sensitivity to hot, cold, and sweets in the mandibular left posterior region. After a sedative dressing had been in place for three months, all teeth tested vital.

Based on these findings, what is your recommended diagnosis and treatment?

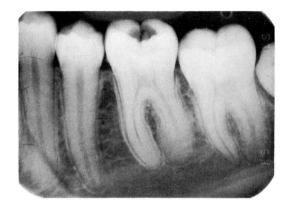

FIGURE 4-144

A 42 year old black female presented to the clinic for a recall examination. The routine periapical radiograph revealed multiple radiolucencies about the apices of the mandibular anterior teeth. The teeth were asymptomatic, tested vital, and were not sensitive to percussion.

1. What is your diagnosis and recommended treatment?

2. What condition is this said to closely, sometimes exactly, resemble?

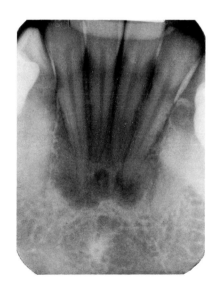

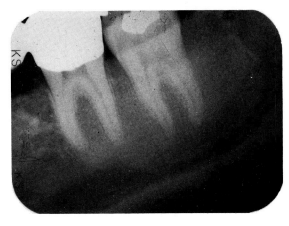

FIGURE 4-145

A 26 year old white female presented to the clinic for a routine examination. The periapical radiograph of the mandibular left molar region is shown. The teeth were asymptomatic and tested vital, and the serum calcium level proved to be 9 mg per 100 ml.

1. Describe the radiographic appearance of this lesion.

2. Prior to obtaining lab results, what is your differential diagnosis?

3. If all other lab values were normal, what would be your tentative diagnosis prior to biopsy?

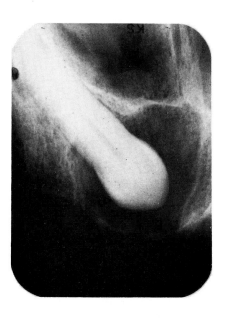

FIGURE 4-146

A 35 year old edentulous male presented to the clinic for a routine examination prior to having a new complete maxillary denture constructed.

1. Of what region is this radiograph?

2. Which tooth is this?

3. What would be your most likely diagnosis of the condition represented by the radiolucency about the crown of the unerupted tooth?

4. Which odontogenic tumor, often associated with an impacted tooth, frequently occurs in this area?

5. What is the large radiolucency superior to the root portion of this tooth?

FIGURE 4-147

1. Give a differential diagnosis of the periapical radiolucency seen in this radiograph of a 34 year old black female?

2. What objective test would be of great help in determining the proper treatment of this lesion?

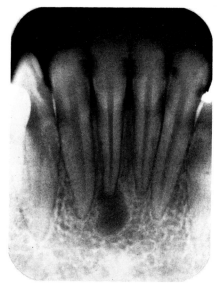

FIGURE 4-148

Is the periapical radiolucency seen in this radiograph the reason for the endodontic procedure that is in progress? Explain your answer.

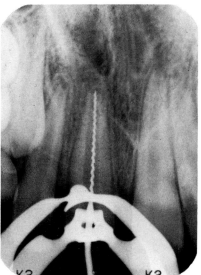

FIGURE 4-149

1. Give a differential diagnosis of the large periapical lesion seen in this radiograph.

2. In the absence of an adequate history and on the basis of this radiograph what, do you suppose, led to the development of this lesion?

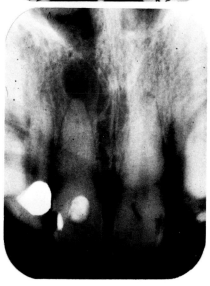

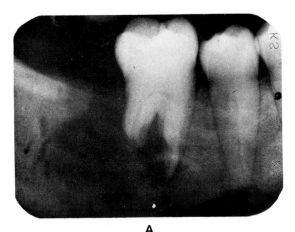

A

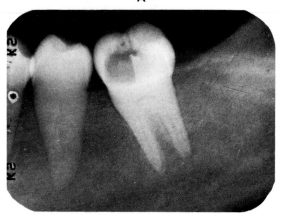

B

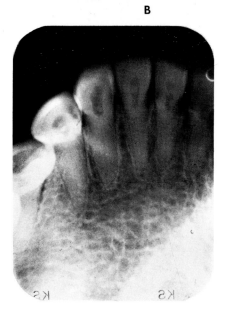

FIGURE 4-150

Lisa Glomer is a 24 year old female who has chronic glomerulonephritis. Although her blood is being dialyzed regularly, it has averaged the following serum values: 12.5 mg of Ca per 100 ml, 1.6 mg of inorganic phosphate per 100 ml, 15 King-Armstrong units of alkaline phosphatase per 100 ml. Histologically, the lesion that was resorbing the molar roots contained giant cells. Urinary excretion of Ca on a low-calcium diet was 203 mg per liter. She had metastatic calcification in some of her fingers, as well as in other areas. What was her systemic condition that produced the changes seen in these two radiographs?

FIGURE 4-151

Janet Thistle is a 26 year old female whose teeth clinically appear normal except for some attrition. Her radiograph, shown here, demonstrates the typical appearance of her condition. Her previous dental records demonstrate that her primary teeth were similarly involved radiographically. When the family history was taken, it was found that her seven year old daughter had similar involvement of both her deciduous and permanent teeth. In addition, the deciduous teeth appeared to be grayish, opalescent.

1. What radiographic changes can you observe?

2. What's the condition?

FIGURE 4-152

Give a differential diagnosis of the small circular radiopaque structure seen in association with the maxillary sinus.

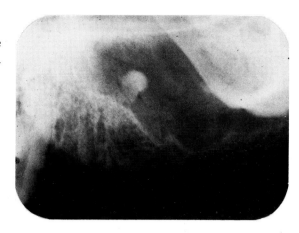

FIGURE 4-153

Approximately 80 per cent of the maxillary sinus in this radiograph appears somewhat opaque, whereas the remainder appears radiolucent. In viewing this radiograph, how would you interpret these findings?

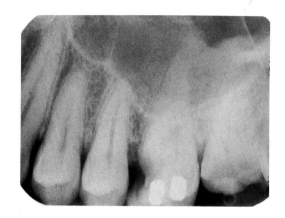

FIGURE 4-154

Give a differential diagnosis of the radiolucency at the apex of the maxillary right first bicuspid.

By now you should know this cold.

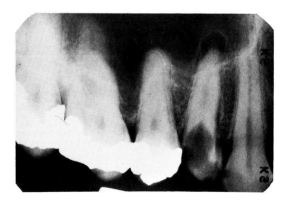

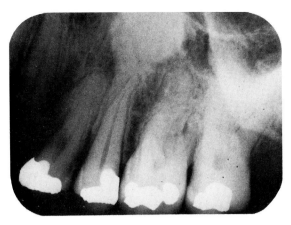

FIGURE 4-155

What is your interpretation of the radiopacity associated with the apex of the maxillary left second bicuspid? The tooth tested nonvital to hot, cold, and electric pulp tests.

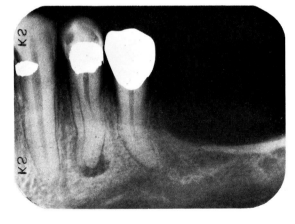

FIGURE 4-156

The mandibular first bicuspid in this radiograph is nonvital.

1. What would be your interpretation of the periapical radiolucency seen in this radiograph?

2. With what normal anatomic structure may this be confused?

3. What notable findings would you wish to pass on to the endodontist?

FIGURE 4–157

Give a differential diagnosis of the radiopacity at the apex of the mandibular first molar in this radiograph. The tooth is vital.

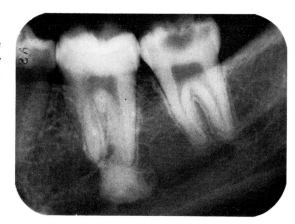

FIGURE 4–158

This 15 year old female patient presented for a routine dental examination. There was some buccal and lingual expansion of the cortical bone in the mandibular right bicuspid region. Give a differential diagnosis of this lesion, keeping in mind the patient's age and sex and the location and radiographic appearance of the lesion..

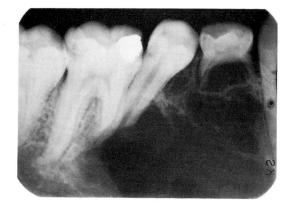

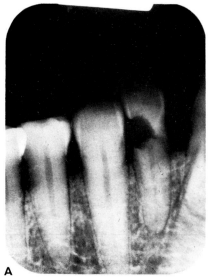

A

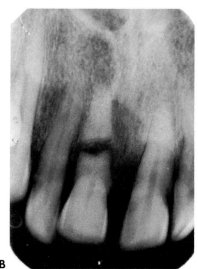

B

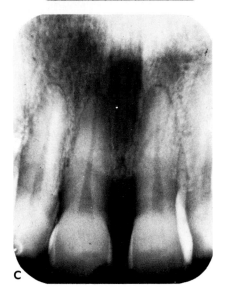

C

FIGURE 4–159

1. What common feature can be seen in these three radiographs?

2. Which of the three radiographs shows a pathologic condition?

3. Which of the three shows a "healed" condition?

4. Which of the three conditions has the best prognosis?

FIGURE 4-160

Compare the radiolucencies seen at the apices of the mandibular first and second molars in this radiograph.

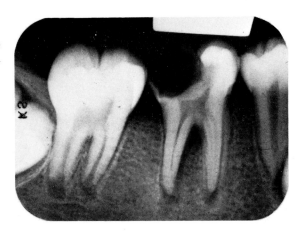

FIGURE 4-161

1. What is the probable cause of the bifurcation involvement of the mandibular second deciduous molar?

2. Can this condition affect the developing permanent tooth?

3. If so, what is this condition?

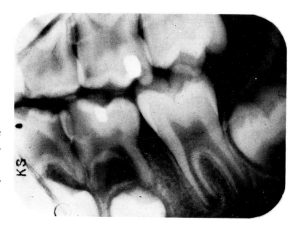

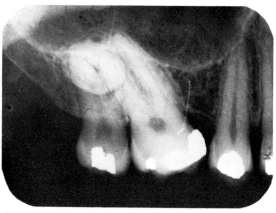

A

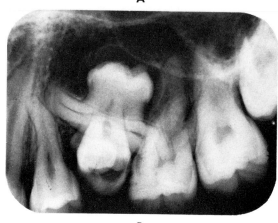

B

FIGURE 4–162

What types of odontomas are indicated by the morphological features visualized in these two radiographs?

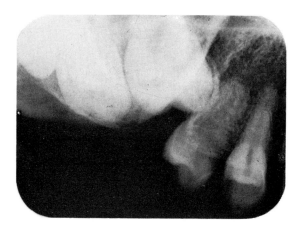

FIGURE 4–163

What unusual finding would you report upon viewing this radiograph?

108

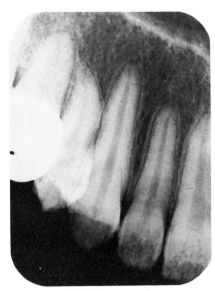

A

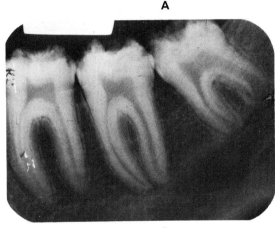

FIGURE 4–164

What condition is illustrated in both of these radiographs?

B

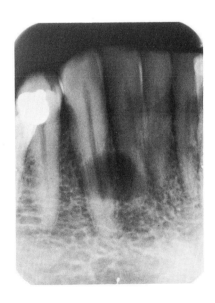

FIGURE 4–165

This 46 year old male patient is asymptomatic. Upon examination a palpable depression was noted on the lingual aspect of the mandible level with the floor of the mouth in the cuspid area. This area was not tender, and all teeth were vital. There was no history of trauma. What condition does this radiolucent area represent?

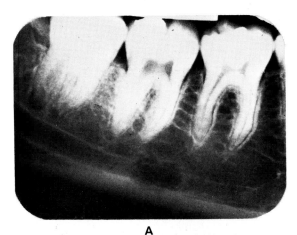

A

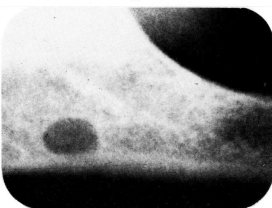

B

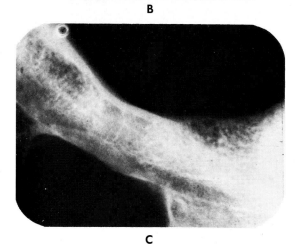

C

FIGURE 4–166

These are radiographs of three different patients. Their findings are considered pathognomonic for what condition? You've seen it before.

FIGURE 4–167

What is the diastema between the lateral incisor and cuspid teeth commonly known as?

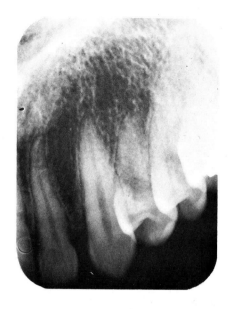

FIGURE 4–168

What is the radiopaque mass surrounding this mandibular central incisor?

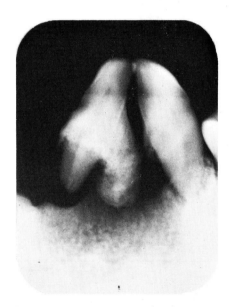

FIGURE 4–169

What are the round radiopaque structures seen in close proximity to the pulp chambers?

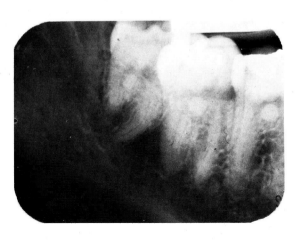

SECTION 5

A SPECIAL TECHNIQUE
USED FOR LOCALIZATION

LOCALIZATION OF OBJECTS OR STRUCTURES

It is sometimes necessary to determine whether foreign objects or dental structures are buccally or lingually situated. A relatively easy method for doing this is called the buccal object rule or shift. It is necessary to take two separate radiographs of the area in question. The first radiograph is taken using the proper intra-oral technique. The second radiograph is taken by changing the position of the x-ray cone. The flow of the x-ray beam is directed toward either the anterior or the posterior. If the object or structure is located buccally, it will appear to have shifted in the direction that the radiographic beam is flowing. If the object or structure is located lingually or palatally, it will appear to have moved toward the source of radiation. Refer to the diagrams.

Diagram 5–1A is an occlusal view in the mandibular premolar-molar area. The dark object is located on the buccal surface, and we can see it in that position.

The periapical view in Diagram 5–1B is of the same area shown in 5–1A. In order to demonstrate the position of the foreign object, merely take a second periapical like the one in Diagram 5–1C. The radiation flows from the posterior to the anterior. Note that the object has moved toward the anterior. This indicates that it is located buccally.

Now, take a look at Diagram 5–2A. The dark round objects are located at the apices of the premolars. When the second radiograph is taken as shown in Diagram 5–2B, the most anterior object moves more toward the anterior. You must realize that the direction of radiation flow is from the posterior to the anterior. The anterior object is thus a buccal object, and the other object is most likely attached to the apex of the second premolar. Well, that's all the explanation you need.

Now that you understand this principle, try the following exercises:

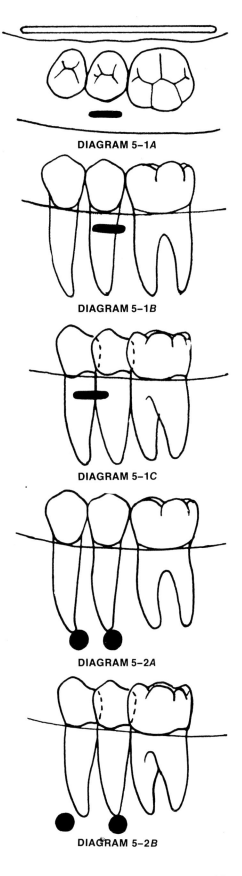

DIAGRAM 5–1A

DIAGRAM 5–1B

DIAGRAM 5–1C

DIAGRAM 5–2A

DIAGRAM 5–2B

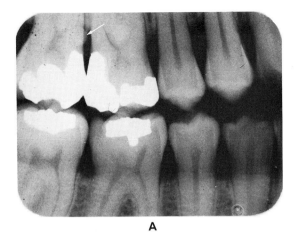

A

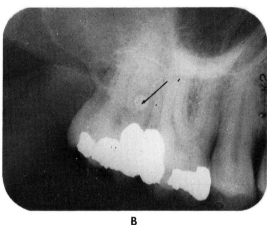

B

FIGURE 5–1

1. What is the radiopaque structure located at the tip of the arrow in Figure 5–1A called?

2. In Figure 5–1B it appears to have shifted its position distally. Is it located palatally or buccally?

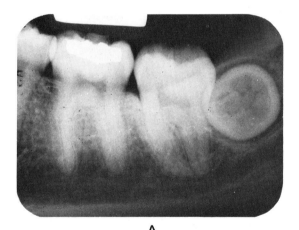

A

FIGURE 5–2

Where is the impacted third molar located in relation to the second molar? Figure 5–2A was taken in the usual, prescribed manner, whereas Figure 5–2B was taken with the x-ray cone directed toward the anterior of the arch.

What's your answer? Remember the rule.

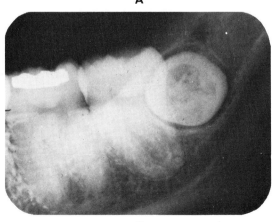

B

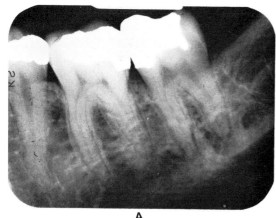

A

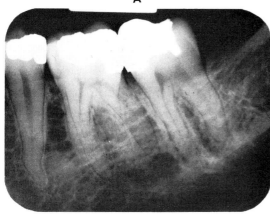

B

FIGURE 5-3

If you look closely at Figure 5–3A, you won't see anything unusual in the root structure of the first molar. In Figure 5–3B the horizontal angulation of the x-ray cone was changed so that the beam flow was toward the anterior of the arch. What do you see in this radiograph? Is it located buccally or lingually?

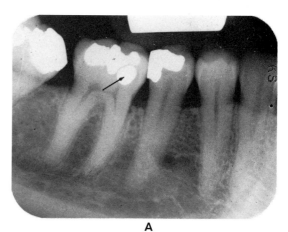

A

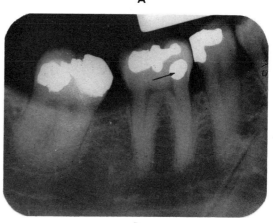

B

FIGURE 5-4

The buccal object rule works not only on the horizontal plane but also on the vertical plane: Here's a good example. The arrow in Figure 5–4A is pointing to a silver alloy. This radiograph was taken using a negative vertical angulation, whereas Figure 5–4B was taken using a positive vertical angulation. Note how the same silver alloy separated from the occlusal silver alloy in the latter radiograph. Is this small silver alloy located buccally or lingually?

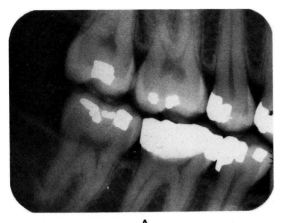

A

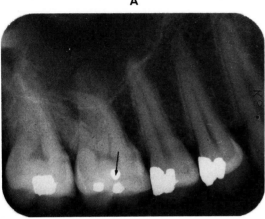

B

FIGURE 5–5

This is another example of the buccal object rule used in the vertical plane. Figure 5–5A was taken at a positive vertical angulation, whereas Figure 5–5B was taken at a much higher positive vertical angulation. The arrow in Figure 5–5B indicates that the small silver alloy is moving or shifting up instead of down. It is moving toward the source of radiation and not in the same direction as the beam flow. Is this small silver alloy located buccally or lingually?

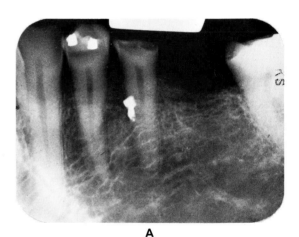

A

FIGURE 5–6

In Figure 5–6A, there is a radiopaque image located over the mesial proximal root surface of the second bicuspid. Figure 5–6B was taken with a horizontal change of the x-ray cone. The x-ray beam was directed anteriorly. Note the change of the radiopaque image. It is now slightly distal to the mesial root surface of the second bicuspid. Is it located lingually or buccally?

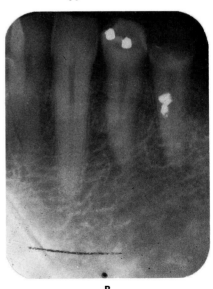

B

ANSWERS

SECTION 1

FIGURE 1–1

1. Maxillary sinus
2. Nasal fossa
3. Superior foramen of the incisive canal
4. Incisive canal

FIGURE 1–2

1. Superior foramen of the incisive canal
2. Incisive canal

FIGURE 1–3

Inverted "Y." The floor of the nasal fossa and the maxillary sinus resemble the arms of the letter "Y," and the bony wall separating the two structures resembles the leg of that letter.

FIGURE 1–4

1. Sinus recess
2. A periapical granuloma, surgical defect, periapical cyst, or periapical abscess

FIGURE 1–5

The nasolabial fold

FIGURE 1–6

1. The nose
2. The median palatal suture
3. The incisive foramen

FIGURE 1–7

1. The nose
2. The nose (peripheral outline).

FIGURE 1–8

1. A nutrient canal
2. The maxillary sinus
3. The cortical plate
4. The maxillary antral mucosa

FIGURE 1–9

1. The zygomatic arch
2. The maxillary sinus (floor)

3. The coronoid process of the mandible

FIGURE 1–10

1. The lateral plate of the pterygoid process
2. The medial plate of the pterygoid process or the hamulus

FIGURE 1–11

1. Pterygoid complex
2. Temporal bone
3. Mandibular condyle
4. Zygomatic arch

FIGURE 1–12

1. The floor of the maxillary sinus
2. The vascular canals

FIGURE 1–13

1. The lateral fossa
2. A globulomaxillary cyst

FIGURE 1–14

1. The nasal fossa
2. Inferior turbinates
3. The nasal septum
4. The anterior nasal spine

FIGURE 1–15

1. The incisive foramen
2. The upper lip line

FIGURE 1–16

1. The nasal fossa
2. The maxillary sinus

FIGURE 1–17

1. The zygomatic process (malar process)
2. The zygomatic arch
3. The coronoid process of mandible

FIGURE 1–18

This is the incisive foramen (nasopalatine foramen). As it appears in this radiograph it could be incorrectly identified as a cyst. Diagnosis should not be based on the radiograph alone.

FIGURE 1-19

The difference is in the angulation of the x-ray cone. In radiograph *A* the positive vertical angulation of the cone is less than that in radiograph *B*.

FIGURE 1-20

1. The zygomatic process (malar process)
2. The soft-tissue shadow of the hamular notch

FIGURE 1-21

1. The external oblique ridge
2. The mandibular canal

FIGURE 1-22

The mental foramen. There has been a great deal of bone resorption so that the mental foramen now appears to be on the occlusal surface of the mandible.

FIGURE 1-23

You are correct if you said this is the mandibular anterior area. The next correct answer is that (1) is the shadow of the lower lip. The round radiopaque area is the genial tubercle, with the lingual foramen showing as a small radiolucency at its center.

FIGURE 1-24

1. The mental foramen
2. The submandibular fossa

FIGURE 1-25

Nutrient canals

FIGURE 1-26

The mandibular canal

FIGURE 1-27

1. The internal oblique ridge (mylohyoid line)
2. The submandibular fossa

FIGURE 1-28

The lingual foramen

FIGURE 1-29

1. The lower lip line
2. The mental ridge
3. The lingual canal
4. The cortical plate of the lower border of the mandible

FIGURE 1-30

The arrows are pointing at the anterior border of the tongue. The film was positioned over the tongue in order to achieve the proper angulation for taking an acceptable radiograph.

SECTION 2

FIGURE 2-1

Adumbration (cervical burn-out). This usually occurs when the horizontal angle of the beam is not directed through the contact areas of the teeth being radiographed. This "off angle" may be in a mesial or distal direction and causes the buccal and lingual segments of the cervical portion of the teeth to appear to be separated. This produces a relative radiolucency that may be mistaken for cervical or root caries. Adumbration may be identified by the radiographic appearance or by repeating the radiograph using the proper horizontal angulation. Clinical inspection is helpful in ruling out caries.

FIGURE 2–2

Phalangioma (patient's finger)

FIGURE 2–3

1. **Cone-cut**
2. The spot on the left-hand side is a clip mark from the processing rack; the spot on the edentulous ridge is an amalgam fragment (amalgam tattoo).

FIGURE 2–4

While the film was in the developing solution **another film stuck to it.** Owing to surface tension between the two films, only one side of the film double emulsion was processed in this area; thus, a lighter image was produced.

FIGURE 2–5

This indicates an **improper horizontal angulation** of the radiographic beam in relation to these teeth.

FIGURE 2–6

1. Failure to place the film sufficiently apically
2. Inadequate **vertical** angulation of the radiographic beam

FIGURE 2–7

By failure to expose the film. This occurs when the time-exposure button is not depressed long enough to make an adequate exposure.

The film can also turn out this way if it is accidentally placed in the fixer solution first. The image is then completely wiped off the film.

FIGURE 2–8

1. **Patient movement**
2. **Film movement**
3. **X-ray machine movement**

FIGURE 2–9

1. **Grainy**
2. This will occur if the developer solution is too warm. The optimal temperature is 68° F.

FIGURE 2–10

Developer

FIGURE 2–11

Excessive curving of the posterior half of the film, which is usually due to excessive digital pressure by the patient as he is holding the film.

FIGURE 2–12

1. **Foreshortening** of the roots and superimposition of the zygomatic arch over the maxillary molar apices
2. **Excessive positive vertical angulation**

FIGURE 2–13

Handling of the film with **fluoride-contaminated fingers.** Contamination from developer solution will give the same results.

FIGURE 2–14

Fixer

FIGURE 2–15

Congratulations—You're right if you said **foreshortening.**

FIGURE 2–16

This is due to **dimensional distortion,** which is an inherent error when the bisecting angle radiographic technique is used.

FIGURE 2–17

Elongation. This error was made either by using inadequate positive vertical angulation of the radiographic beam; or by failing to have the ala-tragus plane or occlusal plane parallel to the floor in the bisecting angle technique and then not using sufficient positive vertical angulation of the radiographic beam.

FIGURE 2–18

1. **Elongation**
2. **Fingernail artifact**
Hurrah! You did it!

FIGURE 2-19

The error is **magnification,** which is rather rare. It is usually seen when the film-to-object distance is increased and a divergent beam such as exists in some short or pointed cones is used.

FIGURE 2-20

1. **Insufficient exposure time**
2. **Insufficient milliamperage setting (MAS)**
3. **Insufficient MAS factor** relative to the patient's bone density
4. **Inadequate development**
5. **Weak or depleted developer solution**
6. **Insufficient kilovoltage**
7. **Expired or aged film**

FIGURE 2-21

1. **Zygomatic arch**
2. Through excessive positive vertical angulation of the radiographic beam

FIGURE 2-22

A **double exposure**

FIGURE 2-23

The rubber roller of the automatic processor. The rubber can actually come off the rollers and adhere to the processed radiograph.

If you look closely, you can also see static electricity superimposed over the mesial root of the mandibular molar.

FIGURE 2-24

This line is radiopaque. Bending the film clinically produces a radiolucent line (see the top left corner of Fig. 2–18). **This artifact is produced in automatic processing machines.** The cause of this occurrence is not understood.

Paradoxically, the corner of the film is bent during processing through the machine. It is bent in an area often folded by clinicians to properly position the mandibular bicuspid periapical view. The ragged right-hand lower edge is an area where the emulsion was torn away from the acetate base during processing through the automatic rollers.

FIGURE 2-25

1. It was **overexposed** to radiation.
2. It was **overdeveloped.**
3. The **developer solution** was improperly mixed, so that an over-concentrated solution was inadvertently produced.
4. There was **a light leak** in the film-processing darkroom.

FIGURE 2-26

Overlapping of the contacts. This error was made by **improper horizontal angulation** of the beam.

FIGURE 2-27

Scratching of the emulsion

Note the film fogging, which may be produced by a darkroom light leak, a safelight that is too close to the countertop, an improper filter on the safelight, a scattering of secondary radiation, chemicals, or the aging of the film (outdated film).

FIGURE 2-28

The film was reversed when placed in the patient's mouth. The tab side of the film packet was facing the beam. The x-rays were partially absorbed by the lead backing; thus the characteristic "tire tracks" or "herring bone" pattern was produced on the film. The film therefore appears light, underexposed, and foggy.

FIGURE 2-29

The lower edge of the film was not placed parallel to the occlusal surfaces of the teeth. Actually, as often happens, the film was properly placed but was moved by the patient just prior to exposure.

FIGURE 2-30

Inadequate fixation. The film was not left in the fixer long enough after development.

FIGURE 2-31

1. Use of **outdated film**
2. **Storage** of the film in a warm place
3. Exposure of the film to **scatter radiation**
4. **Light leaks** in the darkroom
5. Excessive proximity of the **safelight** to the film
6. **Improper filtration** on the safelight for the type of film used
7. Use of **too strong a bulb** for the safelight filter used

You knew these, didn't you? Say "Yes." You'll make us feel better.

FIGURE 2-32

1. **A metal or leaded glass fragment** imbedded in soft tissue overlying the lesion
2. **A metallic object inside a pointed cone**
3. **Scratched emulsion**
4. **A metal fragment imbedded in the bone,** which is the cause of the lesion
5. **A fixer artifact**

In fact, this radiopacity represents scratched emulsion over the superior foramen of the incisive canal. What do you think of that?

FIGURE 2-33

1. *A* – **Fixer artifact**
2. *B* – **Ethiodized oil** used for opacification of salivary gland ducts and some radiolucent lesions
3. *C* – **Shotgun pellet**
4. Other possible causes:
   a. **Air bubble.** With improper agitation the bubble adheres to the surface of the film. This portion of the film is not developed properly.
   b. **Soft-tissue calcifications**

FIGURE 2-34

These are **streaks of developer** from a clip that was previously used in concentrated solutions. Be sure to wash the film-holding clips thoroughly in clean water before reusing them.

FIGURE 2-35

1. **Bent film.** Occurs when the bent corner of the film becomes the leading edge in automatic processors.
2. **The nasolabial fold**

FIGURE 2-36

1. **Zygomatic arch**
2. **Excessive positive vertical angulation of the x-ray cone**

FIGURE 2-37

Reticulation. This is a crazing of the film emulsion due to extreme differences in processing-solution temperatures. The tap water temperature was much cooler than the developer and fixer solution temperatures.

FIGURE 2-38

Double exposure. The film was accidentally used twice to make intra-oral exposures.

FIGURE 2-39

This film was placed similar to an occlusal film and taken at a high angle, so that it resembles a periapical view. When biting on the film pack the patient used excessive force, so that at the points of contact of the teeth the film emulsion was crimped. The radiolucent "lesion-like" artifacts appeared after development.

FIGURE 2-40

Developer splashed on the film prior to developing.

FIGURE 2-41

1. **Static electricity**
2. **Fingernail artifact**

FIGURE 2-42

Fixer stain

FIGURE 3-1

1. a. **Amalgam**
   b. **Gold foil**
2. a. **Silicate**
   b. **Silicophosphate cement**
   c. **Acrylic**
   d. **Composite resin**

FIGURE 3-2

1. a. **Chrome cobalt (or other alloy)**
   b. **Gold**
2. **Acrylic**
3. **Radiopaque cement**

FIGURE 3-3

Porcelain jacket crown

FIGURE 3-4

1. **Amalgam at the apex**
2. **Gutta-percha**
3. **Cast-gold post and core**
4. **Porcelain jacket or porcelain fused to gold full crown**

FIGURE 3-5

Acrylic

FIGURE 3-6

1. **Porcelain**
2. **Platinum foil** (used to plate the dye during construction of the porcelain jacket crown)
   3. a. **Gutta-percha** (left central incisor)
      b. **Silver alloy** pit restoration (left central incisor)
   4. **Bending** of the corners of the film

FIGURE 3-7

1. **Leaded glass fragment embedded in lower lip**
2. a. **Scratched emulsion**
   b. **Metallic object** trapped inside the pointed cone
   c. **Amalgam tattoo**
   d. **Metal fragment** such as a bullet fragment or bird shot

FIGURE 3-8

1. **Six-and-a-half years to eight years old.** The child must be more than five and one-half because the centrals have erupted; he must be less than $11\frac{1}{2}$ years old, because the cuspids have not yet erupted. He must be more than seven, because the laterals have begun to erupt but less than nine because the laterals have not yet fully erupted nor is root formation complete.
2. **Lingual version,** which is apparent from the fact that the bite plane seen on this film is used to correct this condition.

FIGURE 3-9

1. **Stainless steel wire splint**
2. This appears to be a **young** patient because relatively large pulp canals and relatively good periodontal support are evident.
3. **Trauma** to the anterior teeth resulted in loose teeth, which require temporary stabilization

FIGURE 3-10

1. **An ivory rubber dam frame**
2. **An endodontic file**
3. **An ivory #9 endodontic clamp**
4. **Silver alloy restorations**
5. **The tip of the mosquito forceps that were used as a film holder**

FIGURE 3-11

1. a. Lateral incisor—retrograde silver alloy
   b. Cuspid—gutta-percha technique
2. It had an obliterated pulp canal and a porcelain jacket crown.

FIGURE 3-12

Open-faced stainless steel crowns

FIGURES 3-13 THROUGH 3-37

Remember, answers are from left to right.
Figure 3-13—amalgam and radiopaque cement

Figure 3–14—a blade implant and an amalgam tattoo

Figure 3–15—a cotton roll, rubber, and a metallic bite-block

Figure 3–16—a bite-wing tab

Figure 3–17—a retentive pin and a broken burr tip that has perforated, which was used to prepare a pin hole

Figure 3–18—a porcelain tooth, wire mesh to strengthen the palate of the denture, and a metallic pin for the anterior porcelain denture tooth

Figure 3–19—a wrought wire clasp for an acrylic partial denture

Figure 3–20—the maxillary sinus septum (not to be confused with endodontic materials)

Figure 3–21—gutta-percha, a broken file or lentula, and gold casting

Figure 3–22—silver points and a gutta-percha point

Figure 3–23—the tip of college pliers used as a film holder

Figure 3–24—amalgam, gold casting, and porcelain facing

Figure 3–25—an alloy partial denture framework that has acrylic prosthetic teeth that are not visible

Figure 3–26—an alloy partial denture framework, porcelain teeth, and gold casting

Figure 3–27—Eyeglasses (lenses) and the metallic frames for the lenses

Figure 3–28—Porcelain denture teeth

Figure 3–29—Wire (for fracture reduction)

Figure 3–30—an orthodontic bracket, wire (for tooth separation), and an orthodontic band

Figure 3–31—gold casting, acrylic facing (not visible), and calculus

Figure 3–32—a cement base, gold casting, and composite resin

Figure 3–33—metal pins

Figure 3–34—cast gold alloy, a·cement base, and amalgam

Figure 3–35—gauze, a suture needle, and the tip of mosquito forceps

Figure 3–36—porcelain, the metal alloy palate of a partial denture, cement, and an acrylic crown (not visible)

Figure 3–37—a vitreous carbon implant with a gold alloy post

FIGURE 3–38

1. Zinc oxide–eugenol cement-(formocresol) cement
2. A stainless steel crown

FIGURE 3–39

A calcium hydroxide pulp cap and a temporary cement seal

FIGURE 3–40

Aluminum foil that was wrapped around a baked potato

SECTION 4

FIGURE 4–1

1. **Benign.** Notice that the lesion is well delineated by a thin radiopaque line. Malignant lesions tend to be more poorly defined, with more ragged indistinct borders, but this is not a hard and fast rule.
2. **Residual dentigerous cyst**
3. **Primordial cyst**
4. **Biopsy.** This is mandatory, since dentigerous cysts may be associated with or give rise to a variety of odontogenic neoplasms. Treatment, prognosis, and follow-up are based upon a definitive diagnosis. **The biopsy revealed that this was an ameloblastoma.**

FIGURE 4–2

1. Mandibular first permanent molar restored with **amalgam** and a **cement base.**
2. There is evidence of **secondary dentin** formation beneath the mesial

pulpal floor. The tooth is "submerged" with respect to the adjacent teeth. There is evidence of external **resorption** of the roots in the bifurcation area with bone replacement. In these areas, there are no discernible periodontal membrane spaces, so that the tooth is partially **ankylosed.** There is evidence of **osteosclerosis** or **focal sclerosing osteomyelitis** of undetermined origin.

FIGURE 4–3

1. **Traumatic bone cyst.** The age of the patient and history of trauma are helpful hints. Radiographically, the lesion is unilocular and is well delineated, with a sclerotic border at its superior portion. Note that the lesion appears to be "squeezing up" between the bicuspids, with minimal displacement of the roots. Though the lamina dura is often intact, there appears to be some destruction in this case.

2. Pulp test (electrical, hot, cold, percussion)

3. **Surgical exploration.** Usually an empty cavity with no discernible lining is found.

4. **Lateral periodontal cyst, primordial cyst of a supernumerary tooth, central giant cell granuloma,** and **ameloblastic fibroma.** The last two lesions are especially noteworthy, since they also tend to occur in this age group.

FIGURE 4–4

1. **Autogenous transplant** of the developing third molar to replace the first molar.

2. Notice the **flat mesial surfaces** of both the second molar and the transplanted third molar. This flattening was done in order to accommodate the transplanted tooth. Note **decalcification** on the mesial of the second molar and on the distal of the transplanted tooth. On the mesial and occlusal surfaces of the transplanted tooth **caries** is evident. There is an **open contact** and resultant early signs of **destruction of the interseptal cortical bone.** As is common with transplanted

and reimplanted teeth, there is almost complete **resorption of the roots,** and in some areas the remaining tooth structure appears to be continuous with the surrounding bone, thus indicating **ankylosis.** The **pulp chamber** appears to be completely **obliterated.**

FIGURE 4–5

1. **Benign.** The mandibular canal appears to be expanded inferiorly almost to the inferior border of the mandible and superiorly to a level above the mylohyoid ridge. Notice that the cortical bone lining the canal is completely intact.

   2. a. **Anatomic variation.** This is unlikely, since you would not expect a paresthesia to be associated with a normal canal and since upon further examination the right mandibular canal was normal in size.

   b. **Lingual mandibular salivary gland depression.** This is unlikely, since this "lesion," though mainly found in this area, is usually below the canal. The appearance in the radiograph of the salivary gland depression is pathognomonic.

   c. **Metastatic disease.** This is possible, since paresthesia is an ominous sign. However, metastatic disease would not be so well delineated.

   d. **Cylindroma.** This is possible, since this neoplasm produces paresthesia by perineural invasion. This, however, usually occurs in soft tissue containing salivary gland parenchyma rather than in central bone.

   e. **Benign neural lesion.** This is most likely, and three good choices would be neurilemmoma, neurofibroma, and traumatic neuroma.

FIGURE 4–6

1. a. **Periodontitis**
   b. **Scleroderma**
   c. **Early osteosarcoma or fibrosarcoma**

d. **Normal anatomic variation**
e. **Traumatic occlusion**

2. Our most likely choice, in this case is a normal anatomic variation or traumatic occlusion.

Periodontal disease is unlikely since the prominent lamina dura is intact, and also, the height of the alveolar crest appears normal.

Scleroderma is unlikely since the widened PDM space is not generalized.

Early osteosarcoma is a possibility, but usually both sides of the tooth or root are involved. The patient's age, sex, and history of pain would also be helpful in establishing this diagnosis. Clinical observation of abnormally large wear facets and tooth mobility would be helpful.

FIGURE 4–7

1. **Enamel pearl** (enameloma)
2. **Ankylosis**
3. **Osteosclerosis** (bone scar) or **focal sclerosing osteomyelitis** (condensing osteitis)

Note: The first occurs in the absence of infection whereas the last is a proliferative response to a low-grade infection, often of pulpal origin.

FIGURE 4–8

1. **"Submerged" tooth.** This is due to the difference in height between the deciduous and permanent occlusal planes and also to the retention and ankylosis of the deciduous second molar associated with the congenitally missing permanent second bicuspid.
2. **Deep occlusal caries.**

FIGURE 4–9

Toothbrush abrasion. The characteristic features are the sharp, thin, radiolucent line crossing the mesial-to-distal width of the tooth in the cervical area and a distinct V-shaped defect seen in the cervical third of the crown. This latter characteristic can be visualized only when the tooth, film, and beam are exactly aligned.

FIGURE 4–10

1. a. **Attrition**
   b. **Pulp calcification** in the first and second bicuspids
   c. **Calculus** in the first and second bicuspids. (Note the unusual linear pattern.)
   d. **Supernumerary roots** in the first and second bicuspids
2. **Generally indistinct lamina dura** and **horizontal bone loss**
3. **Bending of the film.** In order to accommodate the film in the patient's mouth, the lower mesial corner was bent, thus producing a "fuzzed-out" appearance of the bone in this area.

FIGURE 4–11

1. **Supernumerary tooth bud** and **developing odontoma**
2. **Lateral periodontal cyst**
3. **Retained deciduous root tip, sialolith, torus mandibularis,** and **buccal surface exostosis.**

FIGURE 4–12

Tapered
Easy so far? Go on, there's more.

FIGURE 4–13

1. **Taurodontism**
2. a. **Tricho-dento-osseous syndrome**
   b. **Felty's syndrome**

FIGURE 4–14

1. **Supernumerary mandibular bicuspid tooth**
2. **Gardner's syndrome** and **cleidocranial dysostosis**

Note: The finding of supernumerary teeth does not necessarily imply that a concurrent syndrome or condition exists.

FIGURE 4–15

1. **Cherubism**
2. **Yes,** but not necessarily from this single periapical film. However, bilateral multilocular expansile lesions involving the entire mandible or (sometimes) the maxilla or both may be considered

pathognomonic signs of cherubism. Characteristically, there is thinning of the cortical plates and, paradoxically no tendency for pathologic fracture.

FIGURE 4-16

1. a. **Dens in dente** in the mandibular first bicuspid
   b. **Pulp calcification** in the maxillary first molar and the mandibular first and second molars
   c. **Enamel pearl** in the mandibular second molar
2. **Dens in dente.** These should be prophylactically restored when discovered. The enamel invaginations when cariously involved usually lead to rapid pulpal infection and its sequelae.
3. **Enamel pearl.** These may be misdiagnosed as pulpal calcifications, which can interfere with endodontic procedures.

FIGURE 4-17

1. **Osteogenesis imperfecta**
2. **Dentinogenesis imperfecta** (dentinal dysplasia type I)
3. **Early obliteration of the pulp and root canals** and **relatively less enamel** owing to flaking caused by a defective DEJ. Additional features not seen here are bulbous crowns with narrow shortened roots and root fractures.

FIGURE 4-18

1. **Retained root tip**
2. a. In the cuspid region of the maxilla
   b. **Inverted "Y"**
3. **The nasolabial fold**

FIGURE 4-19

1. **Sialolith, calcified lymph node, osteoma, calcified thrombus,** or **dystrophic calcification** in a soft tissue lesion such as a hemangioma. Do not look at the answer to part 2. That's not fair.
   2. a. By taking a radiograph of the **occlusal view.** This would determine whether the radiopacity is located buccal or lingual to the body of the mandible.

b. If it is not located buccally, the osteoma would be a likely choice. It could be confirmed by palpating the inferior border of the mandible and by biopsy.
c. If this opacity is medial to the body of the mandible, a sialogram would help to determine whether it represents a sialolith or a calcified submaxillary lymph node.
d. If the opacity is lateral to the body of the mandible, a calcified thrombus might be the cause. Confirm this diagnosis by biopsy.
e. In the case of the hemangioma, the finding of soft tissue discoloration is significant. Biopsy may be contraindicated.

Note: In this case, the occlusal view demonstrated that the opacity was medial to the mandible. The sialogram showed delayed emptying time and pooling of the radiopaque contrast material proximal to the stone. The ducts showed signs of sialodochitis, which often accompanies salivary calculi. Final diagnosis: sialolith in the right Wharton duct and secondary sialodochitis of the right submaxillary gland.

FIGURE 4-20

1. **Mandibular molar area.** The clue here is the internal oblique ridge seen on the left of the radiograph.
   2. a. **Periapical cemental dysplasia** (cementoma)
   b. **Chronic diffuse sclerosing osteomyelitis**
   c. **Retained root tips**
   d. **Osteoma**
   e. **Osteoid osteoma**
   f. **Sclerotic bone**
3. Using the radiograph alone, this is a difficult question. The "target-like" appearance of the lesions with radiopaque centers along with the history, strongly suggests periapical cemental dysplasia in the mature stage. Chronic diffuse sclerosing osteomyelitis is possible, however, and has a predilection for middle-aged blacks. It has been suggested that these two conditions may in fact be the same.

The osteoma and bone scar are not usually delineated by a circumscribed radiolucent area.

The osteoid osteoma usually occurs prior to age 30, is often very painful, and usually has a radiolucent center.

FIGURE 4–21

1. **Resorption of the distal root**
2. Pressure during one phase of the eruption of the third molar, which now appears to be fully developed and vertically impacted.

Note: In most cases there is no explanation, and it is simply termed "idiopathic."

FIGURE 4–22

1. **Radiolucent cement** or complete lack of cement.
2. A little cement lining the axial wall of the preparation and secondary dentin beneath this. Showing the characteristic "arrowhead" appearance.

FIGURE 4–23

1. It may be **normal.** This pattern is often seen in normal persons, especially between the roots of a mandibular first molar.
2. It may represent **sickle cell anemia.** This possibility should be investigated until it can be confirmed or ruled out. Sickle cell anemia is known to cause alterations of the trabecular pattern as the marrow spaces become enlarged during the pathogenesis of the disease. One of these alterations of the trabecular pattern is referred to as the "step ladder" effect. Since this pattern is seen in this radiograph, the possibility of this disease must be investigated.

FIGURE 4–24

1. **Focal osteoporotic bone marrow defect of the jaw**
2. By **biopsy**

Note: The fibrous healing defect might be a possibility, but this is usually more radiolucent, more well defined, and often located in the maxillary bicuspid and anterior areas.

The osteoporotic bone marrow defect is often located in the mandibular molar region.

FIGURE 4–25

1. a. **Torus palatinus**
   b. **Osteoma** originating in the antral wall
   c. **Mucous retention phenomenon of the maxillary sinus** originating in the antral epithelial lining.
   d. **Zygomatic arch,** inferior aspect
2. **Mucous retention phenomenon of the maxillary sinus.** This patient is about 12 years old. This can be concluded from the fact that the apices of the cuspid and second bicuspid teeth are not yet fully formed and the second molar is not completely erupted. One would not expect such a well-developed torus at this age. In addition, the palatal torus is usually not so circular in shape. The Waters' sinus view would confirm the presence of a lesion in the sinus. A history of sinusitis would be a helpful clue, since mucoceles are a common sequela of this condition. The osteoma is more difficult to rule out radiographically, and if the lesion persists, further surgical exploration might be necessary.

FIGURE 4–26

A paramolar

FIGURE 4–27

1. **Pericoronitis.** Notice the poorly defined radiolucency seen around the distal portion of the crown of the third molar; it is often seen in this condition.
2. **No.** The roots now appear to be fully formed; thus the tooth's eruptive potential is greatly diminished. Notice also that the tooth is vertically impacted with the crown in slight distoversion.

FIGURE 4–28

1. **Radiation therapy**
2. **Radiation stunting.** The large dosages of radiation required during treatment caused injury to the developing teeth.

FIGURE 4-29

1. **11½ or 12 years,** plus or minus one year. (Notice the open apices of the mandibular second premolar and second molar.)

2. Mesial and distal **retained root tips** of the deciduous second molar.

FIGURE 4-30

1. a. **Periapical granuloma**
   b. **Periapical cyst**
   c. **Periapical abscess** with **secondary antral mucositis.**

Note: This antral mucositis (the broad radiopaque band immediately superior to the antral floor at the apex of the first bicuspid) may be the first radiographic sign of periapical disease in this area.

2. Almost complete regression of the antral **mucositis.**

FIGURE 4-31

1. In the mandibular second bicuspid there is **internal resorption** possibly due to a reactive hyperplastic pulp producing an odontoclastic response. Note the secondary dentin under the distal portion of the restoration and possible periapical involvement. In the mandibular first molar there is complete **obliteration of the coronal portion of the pulp** due to a reactive pulp producing an odontoblastic response. Note the defective distal margin of the restoration.

2. **One should treat both teeth with endodontics.** The bicuspid should be treated in order to remove the hyperplastic pulp before a perforation occurs. The molar should be treated in order to remove the pulp before mechanical access to the canals and mechanical manipulation of the canals becomes impossible. The latter mode of therapy in this situation remains controversial.

FIGURE 4-32

Compound fracture of the mandible
Any questions?

FIGURE 4-33

Mucous retention phenomenon of the maxillary sinus

FIGURE 4-34

Supernumerary lateral incisor

FIGURE 4-35

1. **Amelogenesis imperfecta** of the hypoplastic type involving both deciduous and permanent dentitions.

2. **Congenitally missing** permanent second bicuspid and second molar.

FIGURE 4-36

1. In the **mandibular molar region**
2. **An unerupted molar**
3. a. **External resorption** of the occlusal area
   b. **Complete pulpal obliteration**
   c. Ankylosis
4. By **observation.** Removal would be difficult, and there does not appear to be any significant active pathologic process associated with the tooth or surrounding bone.

FIGURE 4-37

1. The **maxillary molar area**
2. **Sequestration of the alveolar bone.** The cause of this is not readily apparent in the radiograph.
3. The **maxillary first molar.** Remember that the malar process is usually seen in association with the apex of the maxillary first molar.
4. **Probably not.** There is no evidence of a healing socket. This does not preclude the fact, however, that the tooth may have been so severely involved periodontally that there was no socket remaining at the time of extraction.
5. The **flabby, hyperplastic type.** Note the thickness of the soft-tissue shadow overlying the alveolar crest.

FIGURE 4-38

1. The lesion was in the **mandibular molar-ramus area.** It extended inferiorly to the level of the floor of the mandibular canal.

Note: The relative radiolucency seen below this area is the normal radiographic appearance of the angle of the mandible, which is very thin in many patients.

2. **Simple curettage** with incomplete removal of bony and tooth structures

3. In view of the patient's age and the location and appearance of this multilocular lesion with well-defined sclerotic borders, the two most likely odontogenic lesions would be **ameloblastoma** and **calcifying epithelial odontogenic tumor of Pindborg.**

Note: Both the ameloblastoma and the Pindborg tumor may be associated with an impacted tooth.

4. **Yes,** since both of these lesions tend to **recur** and the treatment appears to have been **very conservative surgery.** Immediate surgical exploration and biopsy would greatly aid in removing doubts.

FIGURE 4-39

Mucous retention phenomenon of the maxillary sinus

Good for you. You're getting very good.

FIGURE 4-40

1. a. The **foramen of the nutrient canal**
   b. The **mental foramen**
2. Rapid **orthodontic** tooth movement. Notice that one of the bicuspids has been extracted. The net result is external root resorption resulting in shortened, blunted roots.
3. Obliteration of the pulp chamber in the bicuspid. Note the absence of caries.

FIGURE 4-41

1. **Fibrous healing defect** probably due to loss of the buccal and palatal cortical plates and periosteum during extraction.

FIGURE 4-42

1. A **supernumerary root** on the mandibular first bicuspid.
   2. **Nutrient canal**

FIGURE 4-43

1. Is the **pain spontaneous?** Is there **sensitivity to hot or cold?** Is the **pain more severe at night?** Does anything other than **aspirin** relieve the pain? Does it **hurt more when you are masticating** food?

Note: Obviously this line of questioning may indicate a pulpal problem.

2. **Percussion, hot, cold, mobility, electric pulp test, selective anesthesia**

3. a. **Pulpal involvement of first bicuspid.** Notice the defective restoration.
   b. **Pulpitis in lower first molar.** Notice the mesial recurrent caries and secondary dentin.
   c. **Osteoid osteoma.** If you rule out pulpal pain, this should be considered. This rare lesion usually occurs in young persons and causes intense pain, which is relieved by simple aspirin. Radiographically, it is usually less than 1 cm in size, and has a donut-like appearance, with a radiolucent center surrounded by an opaque border. Notice the apparent displacement of the root of the second bicuspid.
   d. **Chronic focal sclerosing osteomyelitis.** The location suggests possible association with the lateral canal of an infected pulp.

FIGURE 4-44

1. **Paget's disease**
2. a. **Loss of the lamina dura**
   b. **Hypercementosis**
   c. **Cotton wool** appearance of the alveolar bone
3. **Chronic diffuse sclerosing osteomyelitis**

Note: The taking of a head plate might help in the radiographic evaluation.

FIGURE 4-45

1. A **rotated** right central incisor
2. **Pulp stones** in the right central and lateral incisors.

3. **Horizontal bone loss** about the right central and lateral incisors.

4. **Hypercementosis** of the mandibular right cuspid

FIGURE 4-46

This is a **horizontally impacted and possibly migrated tooth.** There is evidence of external resorption, especially of the coronal and apical portions of this tooth. These areas appear to be **ankylosed.** The tooth is located in the **mandibular midline area.**

FIGURE 4-47

1. **Mesiodens** (supernumerary central incisor)

2. **Palatally.** The closer an object is to the film the more radiopaque it will be. Compare the enamel of this tooth to the enamel of the central incisors.

3. a. By taking a radiograph of the maxillary crossfire occlusal view
   b. By varying the vertical angulation (see Section 5, Buccal Object Rule)
   c. By varying the horizontal angulation (see Section 5, Buccal Object Rule)

FIGURE 4-48

Transposition. Notice that the permanent lateral incisor is missing and the deciduous lateral incisor has been exfoliated. The permanent first bicuspid is erupting into the position of the permanent lateral incisor.

FIGURE 4-49

1. **Talon cusp**
2. **"Double" dens in dente**
3. **Prophylactic restoration** of the mesial and distal pits.

FIGURE 4-50

1. The **ala of the nose**
2. a. **Residual dentigerous cyst**
   b. **Incisive canal cyst**
   c. **Globulomaxillary cyst**
   d. **Odontogenic adenomatoid tumor**
   e. **Fibrous healing defect**

FIGURE 4-51

1. **Internal resorption.** A radiographic diagnosis of internal resorption is not necessarily definitive since this condition could also be interpreted as being **external resorption** involving the labial or palatal portions of the root or both.

2. **Acrylic jacket crowns**

FIGURE 4-52

1. The **lateral canal**
2. **Mandibular lingual tori**

FIGURE 4-53

Lingual mandibular tori

FIGURE 4-54

Bilateral impacted or supernumerary bicuspids or both. Notice that the crowns are well demarcated by a radiolucent line that represents the follicular sac of the teeth.

FIGURE 4-55

1. **Attrition**
2. Moderate **pulpal obliteration**
3. **Cementoma** (lower right central incisor)
4. **Bilateral** multilobed **mandibular lingual tori**
5. From the shape of the radiolucency, it seems that the distal of the right lateral incisor has been restored.

FIGURE 4-56

1. **Mamelons.** Remember these from dental anatomy?

FIGURE 4-57

A **double-rooted lower cuspid.** Notice what appears to be a "double" periodontal membrane space. This phenomenon occurs when one root is partially superimposed over another or is seen in bell-shaped roots.

FIGURE 4-58

1. **Enamel pearl**
2. **A pulp stone**

3. The **tip of the nose**
4. The **cementoenamel junction**

FIGURE 4-59

1. a. **External resorption** is present.
   b. There is a **residual periapical pathologic condition** or a **fibrous healing defect** if a resection was performed.
2. a. **Porcelain jacket crown**
   b. Prefabricated **screw-type** core

FIGURE 4-60

It appears to be a **fibrous healing defect** of the socket of the maxillary lateral incisor.

FIGURE 4-61

1. **Chronic periapical abscess** of the mandibular first bicuspid. **Note the fistulous tract and periapical radiolucency.**
2. **Endodontics**

FIGURE 4-62

1. a. **Probably not the central incisor.** Notice the periapical and lateral periodontal areas and the inadequate endodontics. This is probably a chronic situation that could cause some discomfort but not an acute toothache in the central incisor area.
   b. **Probably not the lateral incisor.** Notice the more radiolucent appearance of the crown. This is seen in severe attrition, in which the lingual portion of the crown becomes worn but not the labial. The apical radiolucency has eroded so much cortical bone that the foramina of many nutrient canals are clearly visible. This tooth has probably been nonvital for some time.
   c. **The cuspid is the most likely choice.** In actual fact there was an area at the apex of the cuspid, as well as a pinpoint pulp exposure on the lingual surface, due to the severe attrition. This radiograph was taken just after the tooth had been opened.
2. **Hemangioma.**

FIGURE 4-63

1. **Eight years** old, plus or minus one year
2. **Enamel hypoplasia**, environmental type. The subtypes are classified according to etiology, the most likely etiology here being exanthematous fevers or a nutritional deficiency during the first year of life. In some cases the actual cause may never be determined, whereas in other cases cause is determined with the help of a history and previous radiographs.
3. The permanent lateral incisor, the cuspid, and the six-year molar. The first bicuspid may be involved.

FIGURE 4-64

1. **Toothbrush abrasion**
2. **Foreshortening** due to using too steep or positive a vertical angle or not having the ala-tragus plane of the patient's head parallel to the floor when the film was exposed.

FIGURE 4-65

1. It is not a large **fluid-filled cyst** in the floor of the mouth.
2. It is the **tongue.** The film was placed on top of the tongue rather than under it. This was the case in this radiograph.

FIGURE 4-66

Median maxillary anterior alveolar cleft

FIGURE 4-67

1. **Dens in dente**
2. **Seven-and-a-half years** old, plus or minus one year.

FIGURE 4-68

1. The **incisive canal cyst**
2. **Nasoalveolar cyst**

FIGURE 4-69

1. **Cleft palate**
2. **Peg lateral incisor**
3. The **ala of the nose**

FIGURE 4-70

Diastema. In this area, specifically distal to the cuspid in the mandibular jaw, this is known as the primate space.

FIGURE 4-71

Dilaceration. Note the "double" PDM space.

FIGURE 4-72

It is the **developing third molar**

FIGURE 4-73

Distal drift

FIGURE 4-74

1. During the **first year of life**
2. **Enamel hypoplasia** of the maxillary and mandibular first permanent molars
3. The maxillary and mandibular central incisors

FIGURE 4-75

1. **Enamel hypoplasia** (Turner type) of the mandibular first bicuspid
2. A **microdont** mandibular first bicuspid
3. A **horizontally positioned** developing mandibular **second bicuspid,** which may become horizontally impacted

FIGURE 4-76

Eruption cyst

FIGURE 4-77

Eruption sequestrum

FIGURE 4-78

Amelogenesis imperfecta affecting both deciduous and permanent teeth. (Note the nearly total absence of enamel.)

FIGURE 4-79

1. It is **gold and acrylic.**
2. This is **calculus.**
3. This represents the **mental foramen.**

FIGURE 4-80

1. It is a **benign cementoblastoma.** Note the following radiographic features:

a. Radiopacity is obliterating the root apex.
b. The lesion appears to be delineated by an intact periodontal membrane space in some areas.
c. The tooth appears otherwise normal radiographically.

2. **Yes**
3. **Excision.** This may involve removal of the tooth. These lesions, although benign, are considered to have unlimited growth potential.

Note: The relatively opaque alveolar bone in the upper half of the radiograph probably represents a focal sclerosing osteomyelitis secondary to the periodontal disease present.

FIGURE 4-81

1. **Caries** in the distal of the second molar, the mesial of the third molar, and the distal of the second bicuspid
2. **Calculus**

FIGURE 4-82

1. **Amalgam overhang** on the mesial of the mandibular first molar
2. The **mandibular second bicuspid,** owing to the bulbous root

FIGURE 4-83

1. This one is **periapical cemental dysplasia** (cementoma).
2. This is an **enamel pearl** (enameloma).

FIGURE 4-84

The probable reason for this extraction is **painful pulpitis** (toothache). This may be the cause of the focal sclerosing osteomyelitis present at the apical portion of the distal socket. Notice the intact lamina dura lining most of the remaining socket areas, which indicates a previously healthy periodontal status of the tooth.

Notice a slight interruption of the lamina dura at the apical portion of the mesial socket, indicating an apical periodontitis that has led to a localized breakdown of the lamina dura lining the socket. The tooth was extracted before any further periapical pathologic condition could develop.

It is interesting to note that the distal apex appears to have an associated chronic condition, which is often painless, whereas the mesial apex was associated with an early acute reaction, which is often painful.

FIGURE 4–85

1. Incipient **caries**
2. **Frank new caries**
3. **Secondary dentin** (note "arrowhead" appearance)
4. **Recurrent caries, secondary dentin**
5. **Overhang**

FIGURE 4–86

1. a. In the **maxillary first bicuspid**, there is distal frank caries.
   b. In the **maxillary second bicuspid**, mesial and distal frank caries are present (note involvement of dentin).
   c. In the **maxillary first molar** there is distal incipient caries.
   d. In the **mandibular first molar**, mesial advanced caries and distal frank caries are present.
   e. In the **mandibular second molar**, there is mesial frank caries.
   f. Note the possible redecay distal to the class V amalgam on the **maxillary second molar.**

FIGURE 4–87

Once root formation is complete, the chances of a tooth erupting are markedly reduced. That is not to say, however, that the tooth cannot be made to erupt with orthodontic intervention. Note the apparent ankylosis of the deciduous second molar.

FIGURE 4–88

1. A **retained deciduous cuspid**
2. An **impacted maxillary permanent cuspid** with advanced or complete root formation
3. **Dens in dente** in the maxillary lateral incisor

FIGURE 4–89

1. **Toothbrush abrasion**
2. **Lateral periodontal cyst**

FIGURE 4–90

Peg lateral and **microdont**

FIGURE 4–91

1. It appears to be a **compound composite odontoma** associated with supernumerary and impacted mandibular bicuspids.
2. **Yes. This is done in order to rule out associated pathologic conditions** such as ameloblastoma or keratocyst, which would definitely increase the possibility of recurrence, and to confirm definitively the clinical and radiographic data.

FIGURE 4–92

1. **Nutrient canals**
2. **Calculus**
3. **Periodontal disease**

FIGURE 4–93

1. **Pulp obliteration.** It is localized in **case A,** generalized in **case B**
2. The type in A is often secondary to trauma and may eventually require endodontic treatment. Instrumentation of the canal is difficult and sometimes impossible.
3. The type in B is usually a result of the physiologic aging process. As such, it is not often associated with any future need for endodontic procedures.

FIGURE 4–94

1. **Incisive canal cyst**
2. **External root resorption of the left central incisor**

FIGURE 4–95

1. **Periapical radiolucencies.** The differential diagnosis includes periapical granuloma, periapical cyst, and periapical abscess, as well as incisive canal cyst and incisive canal in the case of the central incisors.
2. **Severe alveolar bone loss** to the apical third of the roots.

3. **Root caries.** The differential diagnosis includes senile caries, radiation caries, and xerostomia caries.

4. **Toothbrush abrasion.** The differential diagnosis includes erosion.

5. **Attrition**

6. **Incisal acrylic restorations**

FIGURE 4–96

1. Amalgam fragments
2. Buccal exostosis

FIGURE 4–97

1. **Extrusion.** The maxillary molars are extruded owing to overeruption.

2. The absence of opposing mandibular teeth causes overeruption of the maxillary teeth. Chronic periodontal disease may also contribute.

FIGURE 4–98

1. There appears to be a **generalized loss of lamina dura** and a "**ground glass**" **trabecular pattern**
2. a. **Fibrous dysplasia**
   b. **Hyperparathyroidism**
   c. **Paget's disease** of bone (osteitis deformans)

FIGURE 4–99

A history would obviously be of benefit. This could possibly represent a **large amalgam tattoo** in the maxillary tuberosity, as well as **some other metallic object** in the maxillary sinus. **In actuality,** the patient revealed that she had shot a .32 caliber revolver into a sink. The **bullet** ricocheted back and struck her in the face. The radiograph shows that the bullet entered at the maxillary tuberosity, leaving many fragments behind as it finally lodged in the maxillary antrum.

FIGURE 4–100

Distal mandibular (pseudo) hyperostosis

Comment: This condition is an apparent increase in height of the alveolar bone seen on the distal of the last molar in the mandibular arch. This may involve the first, second, or third molar. There are two situations in which this condition may be noted:

1. The situation in which a molar distal to the tooth in question has been extracted and the alveolar bone level immediately distal to the remaining molar remains high relative to the remainder of the ridge, and

2. that in which the molar in question is tilted to the mesial. A pseudopocket is noted on the mesial, whereas on the distal or tension side an apparent "build-up" of alveolar bone is noted.

FIGURE 4–101

1. **The tip of the nose**
2. **The upper lip** (lower edge)
3. A **fractured incisal** edge of the maxillary left central incisor
4. a. **Accentuated cingulum**
   b. **Dens evaginatus**

FIGURE 4–102

Hyperostosis

FIGURE 4–103

Probably yes, because of the relatively large pulp chambers whose pulp horns are in relatively close proximity to the surface of the teeth

FIGURE 4–104

1. **Macrodontia** of the second bicuspid
2. A **supernumerary root** on the first bicuspid

FIGURE 4–105

Generalized microdontia

FIGURE 4–106

1. a. **Enamel hypoplasia** of the deciduous cuspid, first molar, and second molar teeth
   b. **Congenitally missing** (anodontia) permanent right central and lateral incisors, cuspid, and first and second bicuspids
   c. **Exfoliated or missing** deciduous central and lateral incisors

d. **Enamel pearls** on deciduous molars

e. Prominent **nutrient canals** in the first molar, cuspid, and incisor areas

2. **Hereditary anhydrotic ectodermal dysplasia**

FIGURE 4-107

Severe attrition

FIGURE 4-108

Calculus

FIGURE 4-109

1. **Black**
2. Older than **40 years of age**
3. **Female**
4. **Yes**
5. **Periapical cemental dysplasia** (cementoma). This condition is in the osteolytic stage in patient *A*, the cementoblastic stage in patient *B*, and the mature stage in patient *C*.

FIGURE 4-110

1. In the **right central incisor** there is an incisal fracture and periapical radiolucency. The tooth probably tests nonvital. Endodontic treatment is appropriate.

2. In the **left central incisor** there is complete obliteration of the pulp chamber and partial obliteration of the root canal. The tooth may test vital to some degree, and endodontic treatment should be used.

Comment: Note the slight periapical resorption of the right lateral and left central incisors. This may be related to previous orthodontic treatment, which is at present in the retention phase with a fixed labial archwire.

On the other hand, this resorption may be interpreted as being a possible sequela of the trauma. In this case, the arch wire was placed to stabilize the mobile incisor teeth.

FIGURE 4-111

1. **Yes.** He has an avulsed and reimplanted mandibular lateral incisor.

2. **Retrograde amalgam in the avulsed tooth**

3. **External resorption** of the apical two thirds of the root of the mandibular left central incisor, with **ankylosis** of the remaining third. The prognosis for this tooth is further complicated by the presence of calculus and its periodontal implications at the cervix. The large diastemas at the mesial and distal are unusual in this area and may be indicative of flaring of the left lateral incisor.

FIGURE 4-112

1. **Fusion (synodontism)** of the maxillary right deciduous central and lateral incisors

2. Probably **not** the fused deciduous teeth. Rather, the developing supernumerary tooth or odontoma superimposed on the crown of the impacted maxillary right central incisor is the probable cause.

FIGURE 4-113

1. It may have been caused by a **primordial cyst** of a supernumerary tooth or by the **epithelial rests of Malassez,** which undergo cystic transformation.

2. **Yes,** as high as 50 per cent within five years when it is of the odontogenic keratocyst type.

FIGURE 4-114

1. **Metallic bite-block**
2. **Gutta-percha**
3. **Sclerotic bone**
4. **Cortical bone** of the inferior border of the mandible

FIGURE 4-115

1. **Developing odontoma**
2. **Yes**
3. **No.** The histologic diagnosis may confirm several other alternatives. First, the lesion may not be an odontoma as such but rather a dentinoma or a cementifying or ossifying odontogenic lesion.

Second, the pathologic report may confirm that this is an odontoma that is associated with other pathologic findings such as an ameloblastoma or even a malignant lesion. All of these possibilities will affect the prognosis, additional treatment, and follow-up of the patient.

FIGURE 4–116

1. In the **maxillary right central incisor** there is cessation of development, with incomplete root formation and apexification; root fracture; and crown fracture.

2. In the **maxillary left central incisor** apexification appears complete. Therefore, root formation must have been completed and internal resorption subsequently begun. There is also a crown fracture.

3. In the **maxillary left lateral incisor** pulp chamber and root canal obliteration is present.

FIGURE 4–117

1. **Painful pulpitis.** Note the thickening of the periodontal membrane space at the apex of the mesial root of the mandibular first molar.

2. Because of **bacterial contamination of the pulp.** Note the microfissure, which is delineated by the well-condensed amalgam that has filled the defect in close proximity to the mesial pulp horn.

3. **$11\frac{1}{2}$ to $12\frac{1}{2}$ years.** Note the incomplete apexification of the bicuspid and second molar.

4. An **enamel pearl** on the mandibular first molar. Do not confuse this with a pulp stone, which is rarely perfectly circular in shape and rarely below the floor of the pulp chamber. Since endodontic procedures are imminent, this is an important consideration.

FIGURE 4–118

Attrition

FIGURE 4–119

Periodontosis. The age, sex, race, and location of the lesions are classic. Note also what appears to be the beginning of bone loss on the distal of the cuspid. This area is also commonly affected. Note the lack of calculus.

FIGURE 4–120

1. **Radiation caries**

2. The **maxillary second bicuspid** (cervical caries)

3. They are thought to be secondary to the xerostomia brought about by radiation atrophy of the major and minor salivary glands within the field of the primary beam. In addition to the alteration in the quantity of the saliva, there appears to be some change in the quality of the remaining saliva that creates a cariogenic environment. Radiation does not appear to have any direct effect on the hard structures of the teeth themselves.

4. a. By proper evaluation of the patient's teeth, periodontium, and attitude prior to radiation therapy.

b. By immediate extraction of undesirable teeth prior to or early in the course of therapy.

c. By patient education and home-care training including instruction on the use of dental floss and self-application of topical fluorides.

d. By frequent dental check-ups both in the early months prior to the possible return of some salivary flow and in the long term because of the ever-present threat of developing osteoradionecrosis.

FIGURE 4–121

Fusion (synodontism) between the deciduous lateral incisor and a supernumerary deciduous lateral. Fusion is the union between dentin and at least one other dental tissue. This case involves two tooth buds.

Note: The distinction between fusion and gemination is often difficult to establish in a definitive manner by radiographs alone.

FIGURE 4–122

Gemination (schizodontism). In gemination a single tooth attempts to divide into two teeth. A normal complement of teeth are present. This condition involves only one tooth bud.

FIGURE 4–123

1. **Hypercementosis.** Note the dentinal outline of the root within the cemental mass.
   2. **Paget's disease (osteitis deformans)**
   3. a. **Periodontal disease**
      b. **Extrusion**

FIGURE 4–124

The difference in the levels of the buccal and palatal bone accentuated by the vertical angulation of the central ray when the radiograph was taken.

Note: This should not be mistaken for a root fracture.

FIGURE 4–125

If you said **buccal mucosa**, you're absolutely right. The film *B* is a view of the soft tissue of the adjacent buccal mucosa. The patient had no history of trauma other than the extraction of some deciduous teeth that had been previously restored.

FIGURE 4–126

1. **Enlarged genial tubercles**
2. Possibly. Note that the patient is edentulous. As the ridge resorbs, the denture flange would tend to traumatize this area.

FIGURE 4–127

1. **Popcorn kernel**
2. **Periodontosis**
3. **Eosinophilic granuloma**
4. **Diabetes mellitus**
5. **Papillon-Lefèvre syndrome**

FIGURE 4–128

Fibrous healing defect

FIGURE 4–129

1. **No**
2. a. **Calculus**
    b. **Horizontal loss of crestal bone**

   c. **Loss of crestal lamina dura**
   d. **Bifurcation involvement of the mandibular molar**
   e. **Radiolucency between the mandibular bicuspids**

Note: The radiograph gives the impression that a lateral periodontal cyst is present. The differential diagnosis of this lesion includes developing ameloblastoma, developing ameloblastic fibroma, developing odontoma, eosinophilic granuloma, solitary myeloma, and central hemangioma.

FIGURE 4–130

1. **Four-and-a-half to five-and-a-half** years
2. **The maxillary left permanent central incisor, lateral incisor, cuspid, first bicuspid, and first molar**
3. **The maxillary left permanent second bicuspid**
4. **Malar process**

FIGURE 4–131

1. A **dilacerated root** on the maxillary right second bicuspid
2. **Mucous retention phenomenon** of the maxillary sinus adjacent to the apex of the maxillary first molar (differential: maxillary [antral] mucositis)
3. An **erupting fourth molar** (distomolar)

FIGURE 4–132

Chronic osteomyelitis of the left mandible

FIGURE 4–133

1. **Chronic diffuse sclerosing osteomyelitis**
2. **None** (as long as the patient remains asymptomatic)

FIGURE 4–134

1. Mesial caries is present in the **maxillary second** bicuspid.
2. There is a distal defective margin in the **maxillary first molar.**
3. The **mandibular second bicuspid** has a poorly contoured distal surface and a slight overhang.

4. In the **mandibular second molar** there is mesial crestal bone loss, markedly prominent periodontal membrane spaces, a periapical radiolucency associated with resorption of the mesial root tip, possibly some internal resorption in the cervical area of the mesial root, and a slightly deficient distal margin.

5. In the maxillary second molar there is a mesial diastema with radiographically healthy crestal bone. Check the mesial radiolucency to determine whether it represents adumbration or caries.

FIGURE 4–135

1. a. The tooth is the **distal abutment** for the fixed bridge.
   b. The tooth appears radiographically to be **ankylosed.**
2. An **amalgam tattoo**

FIGURE 4–136

An incompletely formed **supernumerary root** on the mandibular first permanent molar. (Note the large root canal and wide-open apex.)

FIGURE 4–137

Exostosis or osteoma is the diagnosis. **Excision** in order to avoid interference with the mandibular denture is the treatment. Biopsy is mandatory for confirmation of the diagnosis.

FIGURE 4–138

Idiopathic root resorption
Note: The dilacerated mesial root of the mandibular second molar may be a hint that some transitory eruption problem may have caused temporary impaction of the second molar in the area of the resorbed root tip.

FIGURE 4–139

Amelogenesis imperfecta

FIGURE 4–140

1. **Dens in dente**
2. **Pulpitis and pulp necrosis**
3. **Shallow pit restoration**
4. **The maxillary lateral incisor**
5. **Yes**

FIGURE 4–141

Anterior median maxillary cleft

FIGURE 4–142

1. **Dentinogenesis imperfecta**
2. **Osteogenesis imperfecta**
3. **Yes**
4. These teeth have **susceptibility** to caries about equal to that of normal teeth.

FIGURE 4–143

In the mandibular left first molar caries is present. Alloy restoration would be the obvious choice for treatment. There **appears,** however, to be an **early** benign cementoblastoma associated with the apex of the distal root. Removal of the lesion and, consequently, of the tooth is recommended because of the unlimited growth potential of this lesion.

FIGURE 4–144

1. **Periapical cemental dysplasia** in the osteolytic phase. No treatment is necessary.
2. **Chronic diffuse sclerosing osteomyelitis**

FIGURE 4–145

1. It is a circumscribed radiopacity surrounding the root and periapical areas of the mandibular first and second molars and extending into the edentulous third molar area. The bone has a "ground glass" appearance, and there is no distinct lamina dura in this area.
2. a. Fibrous dysplasia
   b. Hyperparathyroidism
   c. Paget's disease
3. Fibrous dysplasia

FIGURE 4–146

1. The **maxillary right anterior region**
2. The **maxillary right permanent cuspid**
3. **Follicular cyst**
4. **Adenomatoid odontogenic tumor** (adenoameloblastoma)
5. The **right nasal fossa**

FIGURE 4-147

1. a. **Periapical cyst**
   b. **Periapical granuloma**
   c. **Periapical abscess**
   d. **Periapical cemental dysplasia** in the osteolytic stage
2. **The vitality test.** The fact that a tooth is vital is a strong indication that the lesion represents an early cementoma, which, according to current thinking, requires no further treatment.

FIGURE 4-148

No. This periapical radiolucency actually represents the superior opening of the incisive canal, a normal anatomic landmark. The endodontic procedures were initiated as the result of a fracture of the crown, with a pulp exposure. (Note the fractured crown in the radiograph.)

FIGURE 4-149

1. a. **Periapical cyst**
   b. **Periapical granuloma**
   c. **Periapical abscess**
   d. **Superior foramen of the incisive canal**
   e. **Incisive canal cyst**
   f. **Primordial cyst of a mesiodens**
2. Note the obliteration of the canal. This is an indication of a previous history of trauma. The presence of the temporary filling material in the central portion of the crown indicates that an attempt was made to extirpate the pulp. It may be further supposed that this procedure was carried out because the tooth was found to be nonvital. The tooth appears to have been restored very conservatively, and the most likely reason for the development of the periapical lesion was the subsequent development of an anachoretic pulpitis and its sequelae.

FIGURE 4-150

Secondary hyperparathyroidism. This condition is produced as a result of increased renal excretion of calcium, which results in decreased serum levels of calcium. This stimulates an increased production of parathyroid hormone, which results in increased serum calcium. Note that the increased urinary secretion of calcium is a sequela of the chronic renal disease and that unlike the elevated serum Ca levels seen in primary hyperparathyroidism, the serum Ca levels seen in secondary hyperparathyroidism are often normal to high normal.

Note: The "ground glass" trabecular pattern and the generalized loss of the lamina dura. Note also that the more advanced giant cell lesion on the patient's right side (radiograph A) is producing root resorption and extrusion of the molar.

FIGURE 4-151

1. **"Thistle tube" pulp chamber morphology** and attrition (mild)
2. **Dentinal dysplasia type II**

FIGURE 4-152

1. **Osteoma** arising from the wall of the maxillary antrum
2. **Antrolith**
3. **Root tip**
4. **Sialolith** near the parotid papilla. This is unlikely, since the parotid papilla is usually adjacent to the maxillary first molar, which in this radiograph would be near the malar process.
5. **Soft tissue calcification** in the buccal mucosa

FIGURE 4-153

This is often referred to as a **"cloudy sinus"** and in this case represents an **antral mucositis** probably associated with the carious first and second molars.

Note: Infected teeth are not always the cause of a cloudy sinus. The most common cause of a cloudy sinus is chronic sinusitis. Paradoxically, this latter condition may often be associated with odontalgia, and the dental practitioner is often called upon to rule out the teeth as the cause of the patient's discomfort. The presence of fluid in the maxillary sinus may be reconfirmed by taking the Waters' sinus radiographic view and by trans-illumination of the sinus.

FIGURE 4–154

1. **Periapical cyst**
2. **Periapical granuloma**
3. **Periapical abscess**

Note: The relative radiolucent appearance of the sinus is indicative of a lack of involvement of this area.

FIGURE 4–155

It represents **chronic focal sclerosing osteomyelitis** (condensing osteitis). Note the deep restoration and the lack of continuity of the lamina dura around the apex of the tooth.

FIGURE 4–156

1. It is a **periapical abscess, periapical cyst** or **periapical granuloma.**
2. The **mental foramen**
3. a. The **mandibular first bicuspid** has a dilacerated root.
   b. "Double PDM" suggests a possible second root on the mandibular first bicuspid. An additional "off-angle" view is recommended.
   c. There also appears to be some obliteration of the pulp canal of this tooth.

FIGURE 4–157

1. **Osteosclerosis** (sclerotic bone)
2. **Calcified submaxillary lymph node**
3. **Sialolith**
4. **Enostosis** or **exostosis**
5. **Osteoma**

Note: The mature cementoma is not likely because of the lack of a radiolucent line demarcating the lesion.

FIGURE 4–158

1. **Central odontogenic fibroma**
2. **Ameloblastic fibroma**
3. **Aneurysmal bone cyst**
4. **Central giant cell granuloma**
5. **Traumatic cyst**
6. **Central hemangioma**

FIGURE 4–159

1. **Root fracture**
2. **Case A.** Note the large resin restoration, which has weakened the tooth.
3. **Case B.** Note closely the bone that has filled the space between the two segments, and the lack of "reactivity" of the apical fragment.
4. **Case A.** The remaining root structure appears sound and with endodontic treatment would probably support a post and core and crown restoration.

FIGURE 4–160

1. In the case of the **mandibular first molar** there are periapical radiolucent lesions associated with an apparently carious tooth. Note also the bifurcation involvement, which may be associated with a high lateral canal. The bone surrounding this tooth is "reactive," a fact that is evidenced by the indistinct trabecular pattern and the more sclerotic appearance of the bone.
2. In the **mandibular second molar** there is the incomplete apexification associated with normal development of a twelve year old child.

Note the similarities between the two conditions and the lack of a distinct lamina dura at both apices.

Note also that because of the patient's age the bifurcation involvement would more likely be of pulpal origin than of periodontal origin, though this radiograph alone does not definitively prove this.

FIGURE 4–161

1. A **large mesial carious lesion.** It is interesting to note that in deciduous teeth bifurcation involvement as a sequela to caries is the rule rather than the exception whereas in permanent teeth it is the exception rather than the rule. Compare this with Figure 4–160.
2. **Yes**
3. **Turner's enamel hypoplasia**

FIGURE 4–162

1. **Simple complex** in radiograph *A*
2. **Compound composite** in radiograph *B*

FIGURE 4–163

Impacted maxillary right first, second, and third molars

FIGURE 4–164

Enamel hypoplasia

FIGURE 4–165

Developmental lingual mandibular salivary gland depression

Note: When this "lesion" occurs in the anterior area it is not specific or definitive in appearance. The borders are often not well delineated and it may mimic other pathologic conditions.

FIGURE 4–166

Developmental lingual mandibular salivary gland depression

FIGURE 4–167

The maxillary **primate space**

FIGURE 4–168

Calculus

FIGURE 4–169

Enamel pearls (enamelomas)

SECTION FIVE

FIGURE 5–1

1. An enameloma (enamel pearl)
2. Palatally

It should be noted that the radiograph 5–1*A* was taken in the usual, prescribed manner. Figure 5–1*B* was taken with the cone directed toward the anterior of the arch. The enamel pearl appears to have moved or shifted toward the distal or opposite to the direction of flow of the x-ray beam.

FIGURE 5–2

The impacted third molar appears to have shifted toward the anterior of the arch, since it overlaps the second molar. You are correct if you said it is located slightly buccal to the second molar.

FIGURE 5–3

Correct. There is an extra root on the first molar. You're correct again. It's located buccally because it has moved to the anterior with the flow of the beam.

FIGURE 5–4

Remember the rule? If the object moves in the same direction as the flow of the x-ray beam, the object is buccally located. In this case it did, so it is buccal.

FIGURE 5–5

We gave you the answer when we said the small silver alloy moved toward the source of radiation, not away from it. "Lingually" is the answer.

FIGURE 5–6

It is lingual, and we're sure you know the reason why.